WHAT TIME I AM AFRAID I WILL TRUST IN THEE. PSALM 56:3

What time I am afraid I will trust in thee. Psalm 56:3

A Workbook for Anxious Believers

CAROLINE KENT

Counselling with Caroline Kent

Contents

Dedication		vi
I	What time I am afraid…A Workbook for anxious believers by Caroline Kent	1
II	What is Anxiety?	3
III	The Sovereignty of God	7
IV	So who is God?	12
V	Who am I in relation to God?	17
VI	What has the LORD done for me?	22
VII	Journaling : Bringing every thought into captivity	28
VIII	Renewing Your Mind	36
IX	But I can't!	42
X	Fuelling Fear	49
XI	Practicing a Peaceful Mind	55
XII	Treating the Anxious Body	64
XIII	Conclusion	76

Acknowledgements   79
Bibliography   81
About The Author   82

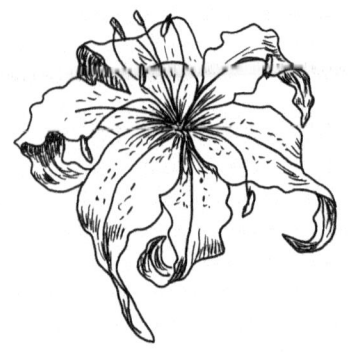

This book is dedicated to:

My husband, Jeremy Kent, who, under God,
supports, enables, and inspires me.

Copyright © 2023 by Caroline Kent

All rights reserved. No part of this book may be reproduced in any manner whatsoever without written permission except in the case of brief quotations embodied in critical articles and reviews.

First Printing, 2023

Scripture quotations from The Authorized (King James) Version. Rights in the Authorized Version in the United Kingdom are vested in the Crown. Reproduced by permission of the Crown's patentee, Cambridge University Press

The images in this book are drawn by Caroline Kent Copyright © 2023
https://www.counselling-with-caroline.co.uk/

Chapter I

What time I am afraid...A Workbook for anxious believers by Caroline Kent

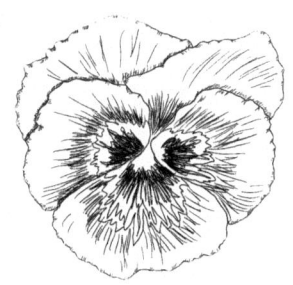

Introduction

This book is aimed at Christian believers who are suffering from anxiety. If you are not yet a believer in the Lord Jesus Christ then, before you can benefit from this book, you need to pray that the Holy Spirit will enable you to recognize yourself as a sinner, who needs to be saved from the wrath of God by trusting in the Lord Jesus Christ as your Saviour. Open the Bible and read the Gospel of John or one of the other Gospel accounts, get in touch with a reformed church pastor and seek salvation today.

If you are already a believer, by purchasing this book and choosing to work through it, you are demonstrating a willingness to bring your anxiety issues to the LORD and to let His timeless truth and wisdom heal you. As with every aspect of our earthly pilgrimage, we must follow where the LORD leads and listen to His voice when it comes to overcoming the trials and difficulties He sends us. We remember with Job:

> Naked came I out of my mother's womb, and naked shall I return thither:

> **the LORD gave, and the LORD hath taken away; blessed be the name of the LORD. Job 1:21 KJV**

Anxieties, fears, terrors, cares, phobias, and dread come in all shapes and sizes. They may have been with us since we were young or may have arisen out of circumstances later in life. The cure is the same. We need to go to the great Physician himself, Jesus Christ the LORD who, through His infallible Word, tells us how we can find peace and healing for our troubled souls.

You may have read the Bible through and through (if you haven't, begin to do so). You may have listened to many sermons on the subject. You may have read many good books, both secular and religious, and yet you are still suffering with anxiety. What, then, does this workbook offer that others do not?

What you will find here is help in how to apply Scripture and to practice, use, and embed it as the foundation of biblical ways of thinking, acting, and living which will liberate you from old, worldly habits of mind which are not serving you well. You will have practice in 'putting on' new biblically based habits, having 'taken off' old, worldly coping mechanisms, following the teaching and commandments of the LORD in practical ways, day after day. God's Wisdom applied and used is what will make the difference. I hope and pray that there is nothing 'extra' Biblical here - no new revelation or ideas of men which are not derived from Scripture itself. (If you spot something – please let me know!)

Workbook

This book is a workbook. It is not just for reading and putting aside. To benefit from this book, you must be willing to engage with and practice the tasks set. We'll call them 'Homework'. The pace at which you work through it will depend upon the time and energy, or ability to focus, that you have. You might read it all through and then go back to the beginning to properly work through it. You might do just a little at a time if you are short on time or energy. Consistency will be key. Work at each set task until you have mastered it, made it part of your daily routine, thought life or prayer life, and keep practicing it, even when you feel better.

Chapter II

What is Anxiety?

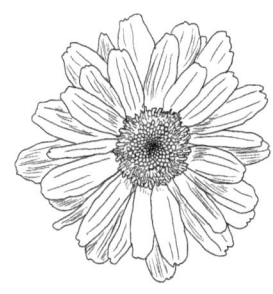

'Anxiety' is a term widely used and often abused today. It is a normal reaction to stress which signals a sense of unease and results in a variety of symptoms. Falling under the umbrella of 'fear', we should be thankful for the gift of feeling anxious in the right proportions in situations that require our attention, vigilance, and perhaps protective action. Without a fear response, we would not notice danger and might react too late, or not at all, to threats.

Where anxiety is a problem is when it has become habitual, embedded or we feel it disproportionately or inappropriately. When there is no present danger, when the stressful situation has passed but the anxious thoughts and sensations remain, or when the sense of feeling anxious is continuous for days, weeks, months or even years, then it needs attention and treatment, because it is not supposed to be a permanent state.

Symptoms of anxiety include:

- feeling restless and worried
- having trouble concentrating or taking in information (brain fog)
- temperature fluctuations (hot, sweaty, cold, clammy)
- dizziness, nausea
- heart palpitations,
- shortness of breath
- insomnia / oversleeping / exhaustion
- panic / spinning thoughts / mind blanks
- vivid nightmares / night terrors
- loss of appetite / overeating
- a sense of impending doom

- flashbacks of traumatic events

You may experience all of these occasionally, that's normal, but if you are regularly experiencing four or more of these symptoms, and they are recurring and lasting several weeks or months, do not ignore them and just hope they go away. Get a check up with a medical professional, talk to your pastor, elders or trusted church members and seek to apply scriptural truth to address the symptoms.

If your life circumstances are perpetuating the problem (illness, relationship problems, financial worries, loneliness etc.) do not wait for 'things to be better' before addressing the anxiety symptoms. Circumstances may or may not change for the better, but you can, regardless, arm yourself with helpful, scripturally based principles and practices which will help you cope with whatever you are dealing with.

If you are suffering with ongoing anxiety, it is highly likely that you are trying to cope in your own strength. Don't! Instead, remember that the Lord Jesus Christ said:

> These things I have spoken unto you, that in me ye might have peace. In the world ye shall have tribulation: but be of good cheer; I have overcome the world. John 16:33 KJV

Learn how to seek the LORD in all your trials and feel peace instead of anxiety. Learn how to have confidence in the power of His might and His promises in the face of life's difficulties.

Now write down your experience with anxiety: symptoms, duration, causes, and circumstances.

Journal

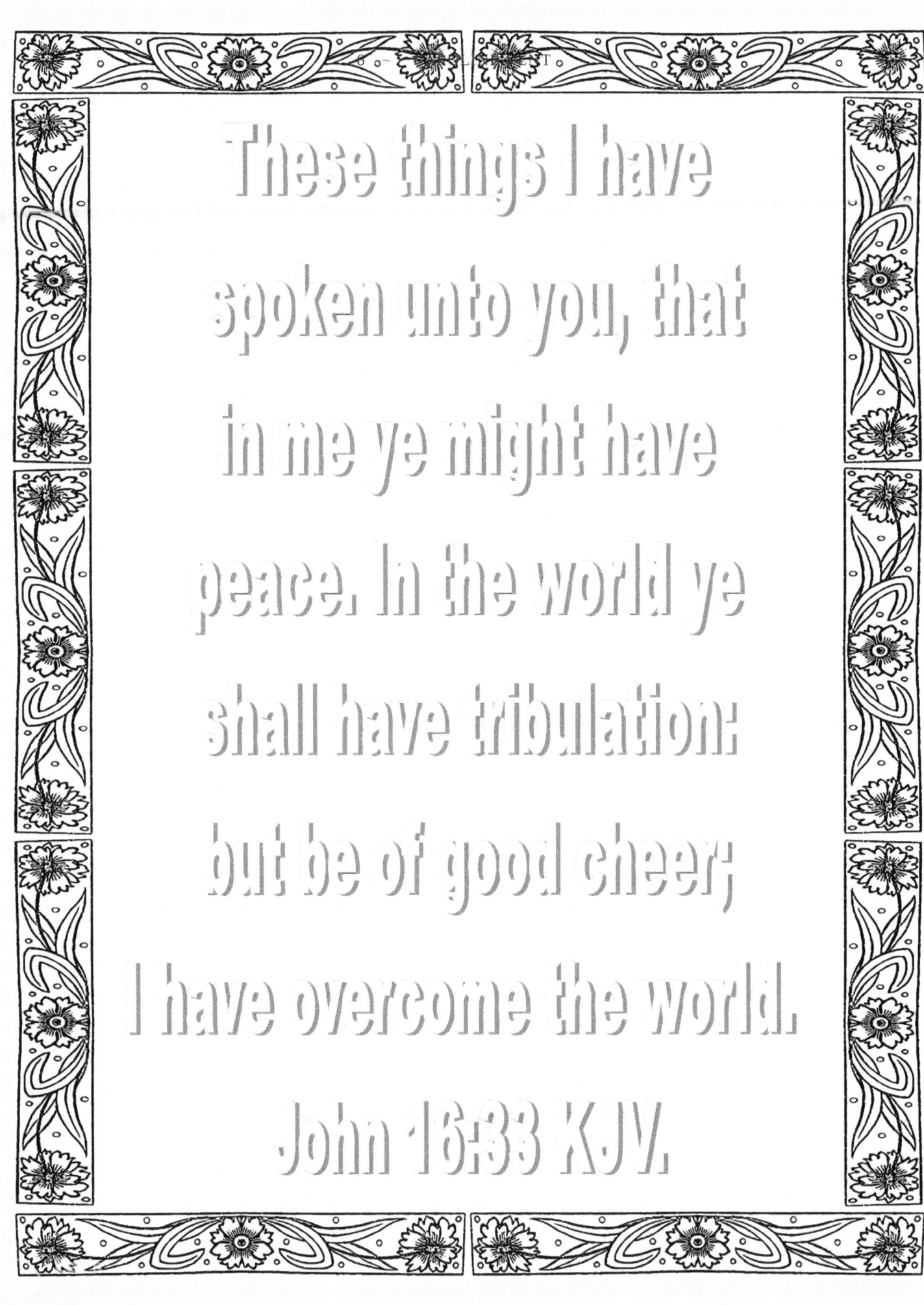

These things I have spoken unto you, that in me ye might have peace. In the world ye shall have tribulation: but be of good cheer; I have overcome the world. John 16:33 KJV.

Chapter III

The Sovereignty of God

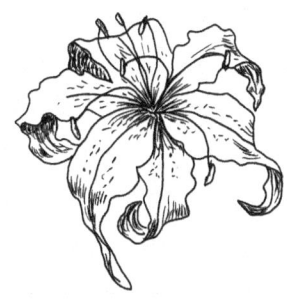

The first and most important step is to address your thinking and understanding about just who and what God is.

In our anxiety, we are often focused on 'the problem' or 'my feelings' or 'how can I get through today?' We are approaching life as if we are alone and independent, having to draw upon our own personal resources, having to force ourselves to put one step in front of the other as if there was no one and nothing but our own will power to get us through.

Stop.

This is not a true assessment of the situation.

You may be thinking, "I know what you are going to say, but I have prayed, I have asked God for help, He doesn't seem to be listening or answering."

I hope you have prayed and keep praying, but just who are you praying to? On the journal page below, write down who or what is in your mind when you pray. Be honest. Don't write what you think the right answer is.

Write about the reality of what you are thinking about the God to whom you are praying.

Journal

And now, write about what you think God thinks of you. What is your relationship with Him? Again, be brutally honest. This is key.

Usually, we either have an unscriptural understanding of who God is, or we have a faulty view of who we are in relation to God, or both!

The result of this is that we don't know how to have a helpful, healing, strengthening and empowering prayer life or relationship with Almighty God. We don't know how to apply the many wonderful promises in the Scriptures to our personal circumstances. We don't know how to see ourselves and our lives in the context of the Gospel of Jesus Christ or to receive wisdom from the Holy Spirit through the Scriptures. If our beliefs are incorrect, unbalanced, or unapplied, they are no good to us. We need a biblically accurate faith, applied.

We need to stop living as 'functional atheists', behaving as if God is not omnipresent, omnipotent, and graciously, mercifully interested in His children and *every* aspect of their lives.

Journal

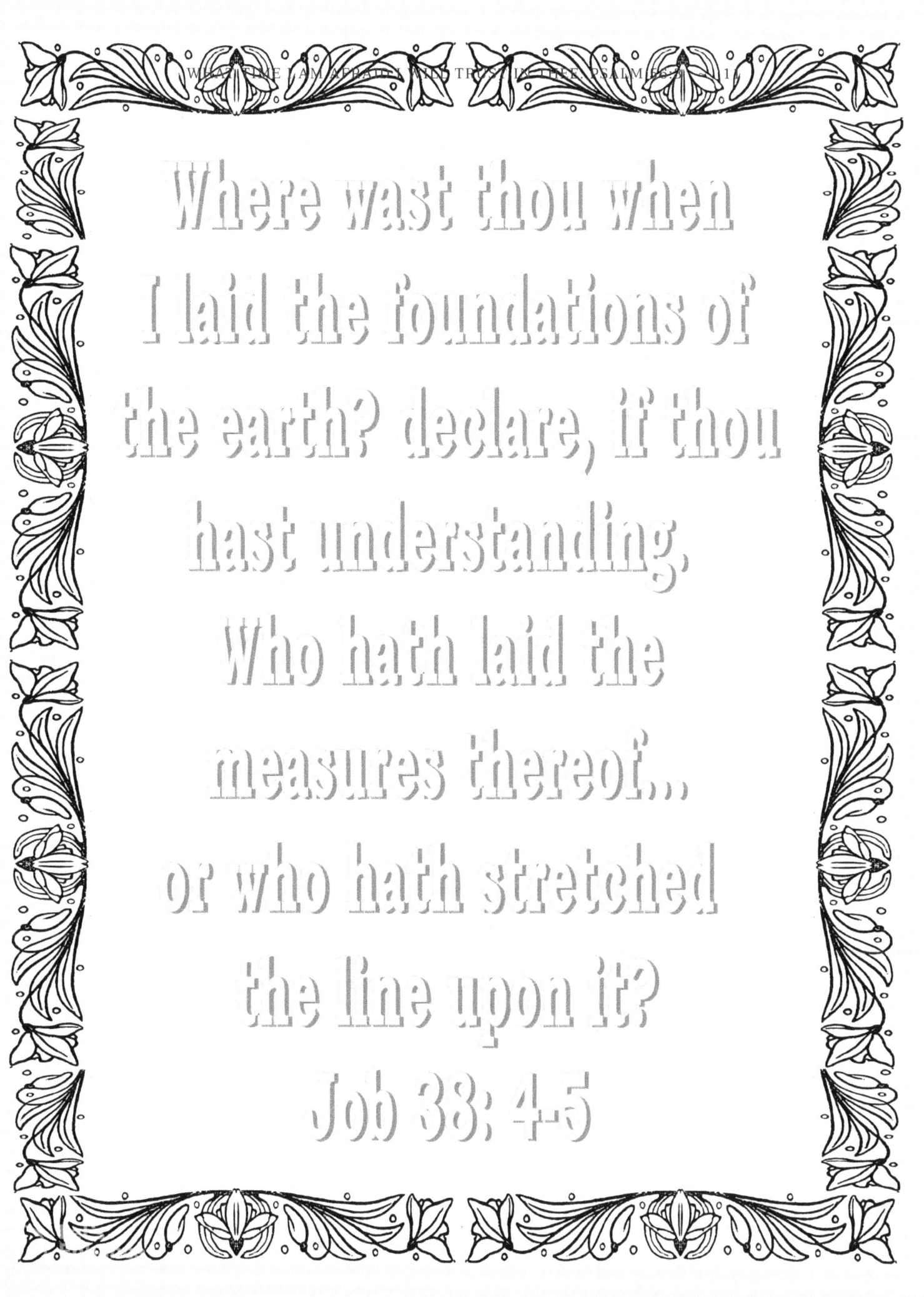

Where wast thou when I laid the foundations of the earth? declare, if thou hast understanding, Who hath laid the measures thereof... or who hath stretched the line upon it? Job 38: 4-5

Chapter IV

So who is God?

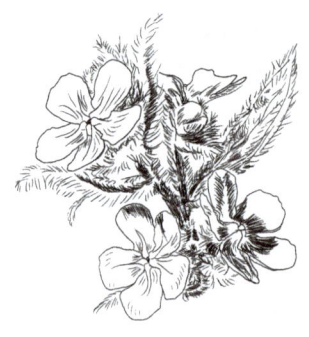

Theologians have been trying to define God, as He reveals Himself in the pages of Scripture, since the early church. After the protestant reformation, when many more scholars had access to the Bible in the original Greek and Hebrew, groups of 'divines' (biblical scholars, ministers of the word and ordained pastors) sought to produce a definitive 'confession of faith' around which the church could come to agreement and could use to teach and guide their flocks. The Westminster Confession is one of these, and is highly respected and widely used among reformed churches. The following quote is, in the original, linked to multiple Scripture texts which support each statement.

The Westminster Confession (1647) states:

> *"There is but one only living and true God, who is infinite in being and perfection, a most pure spirit, invisible, without body, parts, or passions; immutable, immense, eternal, incomprehensible, almighty, most wise, most holy, most free, most absolute, working all things according to the counsel of His own immutable and most righteous will, for His own glory; most loving, gracious, merciful, long-suffering, abundant in goodness and truth, forgiving iniquity, transgression, and sin, the rewarder of them that diligently seek Him; and withal, most just, and terrible in His judgments; hating all sin, and who will by no means clear the guilty." The Westminster Confession of Faith (Ligonier.org)*[1]

Now, that's a lot to try and hold in our minds! But try we must because, when we stray from this definition, we begin to re-imagine God according to human proportions, attitudes, and responses if we are not careful. We shrink the LORD and strip Him of His attributes, thus rendering Him a false idol which will do us no good. This is what was happening to Job toward the end of his trials. He was forgetting just who God really is. So, the LORD, graciously and pointedly reminds him!

> Where wast thou when I laid the foundations of the earth? declare, if thou hast understanding. Job 38:4 KJV

The LORD God speaks to a desperately unhappy Job, out of the whirlwind. We might have expected words of comfort after all Job's losses and trials, but no, instead, the LORD asks him a question and challenges him!

What is God doing here? With perfect precision, the LORD gets to the heart of Job's problem. Job has forgotten who he is talking to, the Sovereign LORD God, maker of heaven and earth, sustainer of all things, infallible, immutable, the only wise God. Job, together with his 'comforters,' have been trying to comprehend the ways and workings of God in human terms. They have been trying to grapple with eternal and transcendent realities with their finite minds. The first action of the suffering Christian should be to come humbly before Almighty God and recognize His sovereignty. He is a vastly greater being than we can even imagine, and remember, He knows what He is doing!

Have we fallen into praying for God to fix our situation according to our own design? Or worse, praying to a god of our own design?

When our lives are in seeming chaos, our stresses seem beyond our ability and energy to cope with, we can tend to look to God to 'solve' our situation in the way that we desire. We want explanations, answers, a plan of action, a quick fix or total cure. In our distress, like Job, we might even wish we had never been born or were no longer alive to have to deal with all that is in front of us.

God answers our earth-bound, human desires by lifting our eyes up and beyond the immediate to the eternal, Himself. Neither Job nor we have any right to make demands of God. He is our maker, our sustainer and the provider of life and breath every moment of every day of our lives. It is only by His will that we exist at all.

> It is of the LORD's mercies that we are not consumed, because his compassions fail not. Lamentations 3:22 KJV

Job has been trying to tell God what God ought to do about His situation. The LORD answers:

> Shall he that contendeth with the Almighty instruct him? he that reproveth God, let him answer it. Job 40:2 KJV

With Job, our response should be,

> Behold, I am vile; what shall I answer thee? I will lay mine hand upon my mouth. Job 40:4 KJV

When our situation or feelings overwhelm us, we should spend time remembering that our great God knows exactly what is going on, what we are going through and how He will bring us through it. He has planned and decreed all that we are experiencing and knows where it will take us in both time and eternity.

Submitting to God's will and God's way, seeing our lives in the light of the enormity and magnificence of who God is, is the first step to relieving our anxiety. If God is really, absolutely in control, expending unnecessary energy worrying, being fearful or anxious, makes little sense. We can and should trust God to be in charge and in control of all things. If indeed He is, then we don't have to be! We can rest in and trust in His judgement and promises.

Our fear (awe, respect, adoration, trembling astonishment), should be focused on the LORD rather than on earthly situations or people:

> And I say unto you my friends, Be not afraid of them that kill the body, and after that have no more that they can do. But I will forewarn you whom ye shall fear: Fear him, which after he hath killed hath power to cast into hell; yea, I say unto you, Fear him. Are not five sparrows sold for two farthings, and not one of them is forgotten before God? But even the very hairs of your head are all numbered. Fear not therefore: ye are of more value than many sparrows. Also I say unto you, Whosoever shall confess me before men, him shall the Son of man also confess before the angels of God: But he that denieth me before men shall be denied before the angels of God. Luke 12:4-9 KJV

A study of one of the historic confessions would be very valuable if you have the time. The Westminster Confession[2], the 1689 Baptist Confession[3], and other reformed confessions which arose from the Reformation each carefully set out the foundational beliefs we should have, drawn from the Scriptures. (Note, there are some denominational differences around baptism and Church government in particular.)

Further reading, if you have time:

The Sovereignty of God[4] and *The Attributes of God*[5] by Arthur W Pink, both available on the Monergism.com[6] website.

> *HOMEWORK*
>
> Colour the following page, carefully, prayerfully, a little each day for this week. As you do, let your mind dwell upon the attributes and excellencies of our Holy God. In this vision of Isaiah, the seraphim cry out in praise of God and Isaiah is terrified by the glory of the LORD. Learn the verse as you colour. Consider the magnitude of the LORD and how everything around you points to His glory. Read and re-read the extract from the Westminster Confession. Pray, praise, and worship the LORD.
>
> Why colouring? When our hands and eyes are busily focussed on a practical task, it frees our minds to focus on the truth we are seeking to learn and embed. Doing the task carefully and beautifully will help to emphasize the importance of carefully considering who God is when we pray to Him.
>
> *PRAYER*
>
> Sovereign LORD God, maker of heaven and earth, sustainer, provider and only Saviour of sinners, give me a biblical understanding of your greatness, as much as my finite and sinful mind can comprehend. Help me to trust in your power, wisdom and might and in your love for your blood-bought children. In Jesus's precious name, Amen.

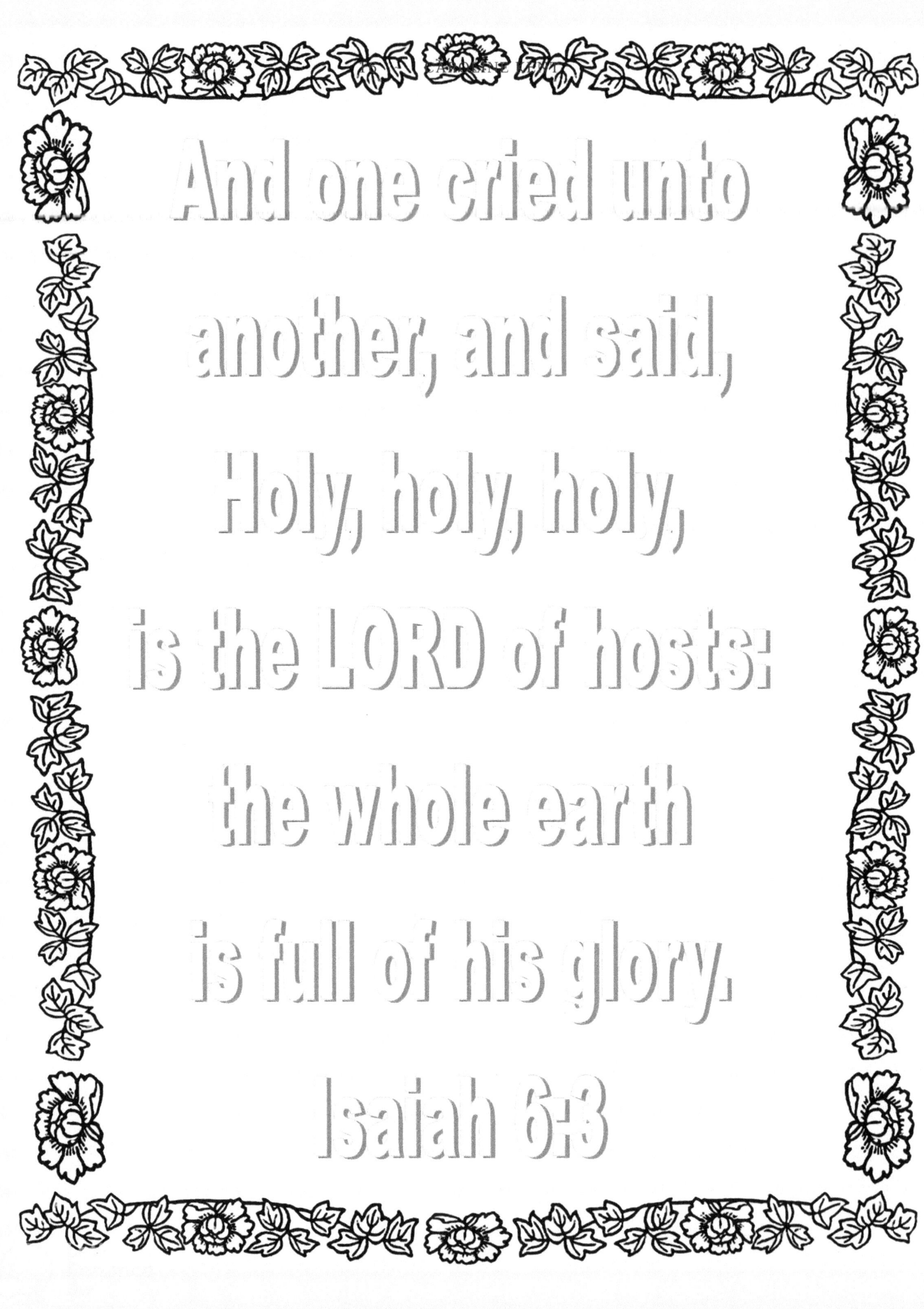

And one cried unto another, and said, Holy, holy, holy, is the LORD of hosts: the whole earth is full of his glory. Isaiah 6:3

Chapter V

Who am I in relation to God?

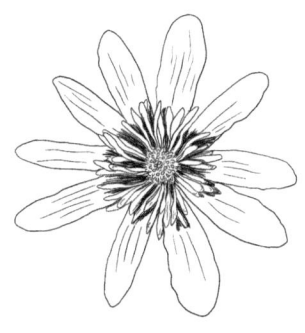

John Gill (1697 – 1771), commenting on Psalm 139, says,

"...the formation of man is not of himself, nor of his parents, but of God, and is very wonderful in all its parts; it has been matter of astonishment to many...marvellous are [God's] works; of creation, providence, sustentation of all creatures, the government of the world, the redemption of mankind, the work of grace and conversion, the perseverance of the saints, and their eternal salvation." (Biblehub.com)[7]

Matthew Henry (1662 – 1714) remarks, *"No veil can hide us from God; not the thickest darkness. No disguise can save any person or action from being seen in the true light by him...On the other hand, the believer cannot be removed from the supporting, comforting presence of his Almighty Friend."* (Biblehub.com)[8]

The magnificence and yet imminence of God is demonstrated in the way in which He has woven human beings into existence, sustains them and knows them each intimately.

Read the whole of Psalm 139, carefully, prayerfully.

But be honest, how are you in the habit of thinking about yourself? How would you describe yourself when you think about who and what you are?

Write down what you *do* think not what you think you *should* think!

Journal

Do you live from day to day, remembering that you are fearfully and wonderfully made, and that God is always with you and knows everything about you? Or do you live as if He was absent, and you were alone in the world? A world that you believe has it in for you or judges you and finds you wanting by their standard? Do you fear that God wants nothing to do with you? That you are too small, too insignificant, that you do not matter to the great I AM?

Your habitual way of thinking about yourself is important. Is it true, though, and is it biblical?

If the LORD has begun that good work in you, you should be able to sing with Solomon,

> I am my beloved's, and my beloved is mine: he feedeth among the lilies.
> Song of Solomon 6:3 KJV

You should know yourself to be part of that great vine and that you abide in Christ and He in you, that you are there with all the body of Christ, loved and abiding in love (John 15). You should know yourself to be redeemed by the blood of Jesus Christ, adopted into the very family of God as an heir, able to call God, "Abba, Father" (Galatians 4:1-7).

In Christ we have become new creatures (2 Corinthians 5:17), no longer in bondage to sin, no longer destined for eternal judgement, reconciled and at peace with God.

Perhaps you say in your heart, 'Yes, but...I don't feel that way!' How you *feel* doesn't alter the truth as it is in Scripture. How you *feel* doesn't change what Christ has done. Distinguishing between biblical *fact* and personal *feeling* is going to be very important.

Perhaps you have bought the lie that to be 'okay' you have to be a strong, self-confident, independent person who is successful, beautiful, athletic, popular? Getting a biblical understanding of ourselves in relation to God as opposed to the one imposed by modern humanistic society is essential.

How we understand ourselves in relation to our God is far more important than what society thinks. We should be dependent, submissive, reverent, adoring, deriving our value and worth from the value and worth of the Lord Jesus Christ and the fact that the LORD has shown us grace and mercy.

If you have sin-laden, world-soaked, devil-influenced views of yourself, these need to be weeded out and replaced with the beautiful, astonishing, liberating truths about what the Lord Jesus Christ has changed you into.

> I will praise thee; for I am fearfully and wonderfully made: marvellous are thy works; and that my soul knoweth right well.
> My substance was not hid from thee, when I was made in secret, and curiously wrought in the lowest parts of the earth.
> Thine eyes did see my substance, yet being unperfect; and in thy book all my members were written, which in continuance were fashioned, when as yet there was none of them.
> How precious also are thy thoughts unto me, O God! how great is the sum of them!
> If I should count them, they are more in number than the sand: when I awake, I am still with thee.
> Psalm 139:14-18 KJV

HOMEWORK

Overcoming habitual ways of thinking takes time and effort. As you colour the next page, keep telling yourself truths about yourself as you are in the Lord Jesus Christ. Not how you feel or imagine yourself to be, but what Scripture says and how beloved you are to the LORD because you are one of His redeemed people.

Feelings-led thinking can quickly lead us astray. We need to challenge those thoughts that are contrary to scriptural teaching and those 'gut feelings' that feel so 'right' but are contrary to God's Word and Truth.

PRAYER

Confession and repentance if you have been applying an unbiblical understanding of God or of yourself in relation to God. Prayer for change and the ability to hold right beliefs and apply them in your daily walk and prayer life.

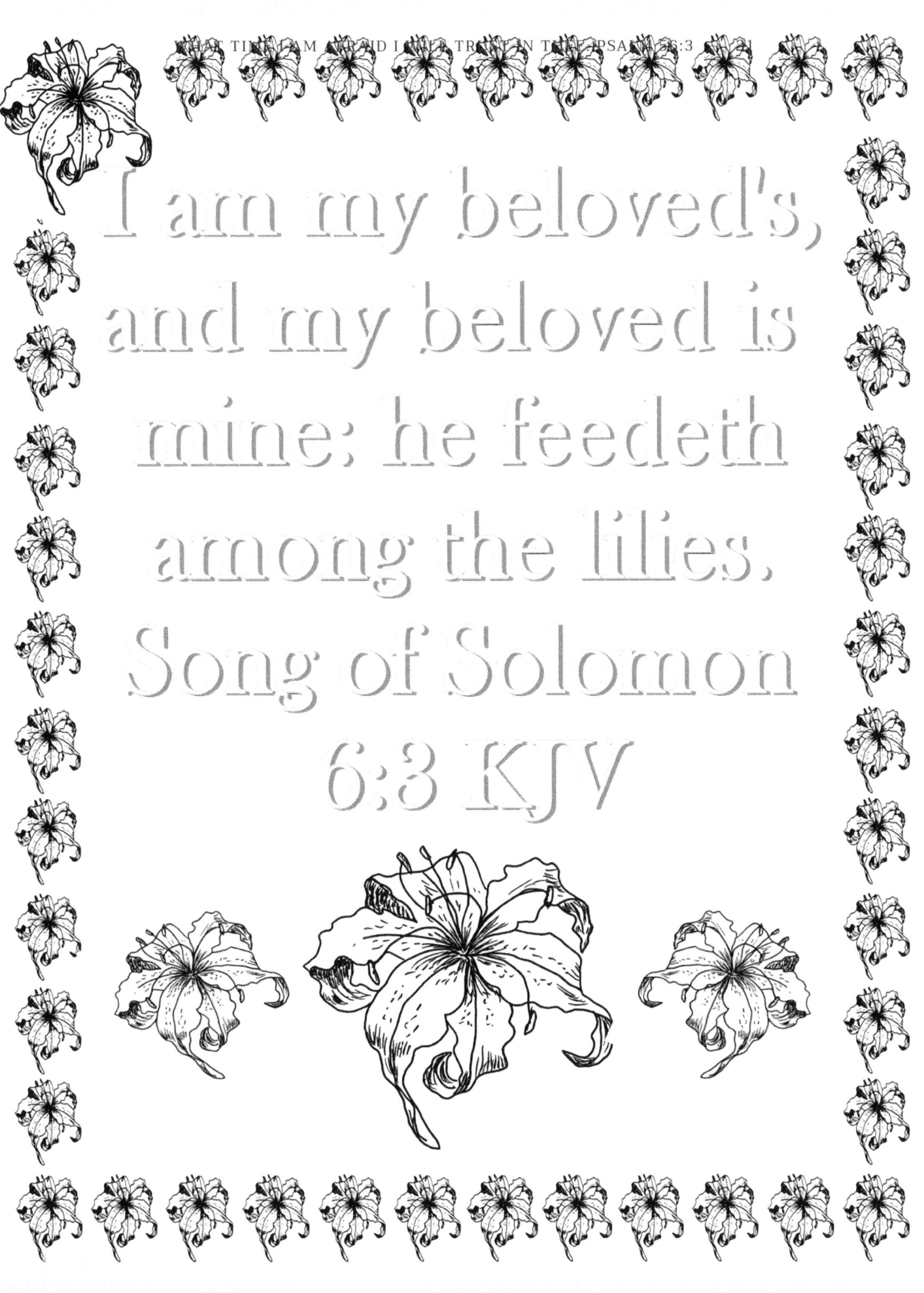

Chapter VI

What has the LORD done for me?

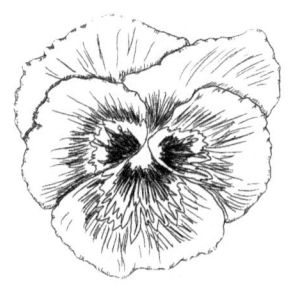

To consolidate your knowledge (rather than feeling) about your identity in Christ, it is always helpful to remember, study and rehearse what the LORD has, in fact, done for you. You will find this principle in the Psalms. The psalmist will often cry out in anguish, express his difficulty to the LORD and seek His aid. Then he will rehearse all the ways in which God has helped him in the past. This reassures him and gives him confidence that the LORD will help in the future.

For some people there is a great contrast between before they were saved and after. They can see that the LORD has worked amazingly in their lives.

> He brought me up also out of an horrible pit, out of the miry clay, and set my feet upon a rock, and established my goings. Psalm 40:2 KJV

Some people cannot pinpoint the day or hour of their conversion, it was a slow process, perhaps, over years. Maybe living in a Christian family or always having had a sense of God in your life, but not dramatically, you understand that:

> He maketh me to lie down in green pastures: he leadeth me beside the still waters. Psalm 23:2 KJV

Regardless of the manner of your salvation, the LORD has mercifully rescued you from the judgement that we all deserve through the suffering and sacrifice of His only begotten Son and (if that wasn't enough), kept you, given you breath each day, supplied your needs, brought you under the ministry of the Word, enabled you to read the Bible, given you life skills, placed you in His family the church, and is sanctifying you and fitting you for an eternal home in glory as a co-heir with Christ!

You are or will be:

- **Elect** & **effectually called**
- **Regenerate**: born again of the Holy Spirit
- **Converted**: the recipient of saving faith
- **Justified** & enabled to **repent**, freed from the bondage of sin & clothed in Christ's righteousness
- **Adopted** into the family of God
- **Sanctified**: able to do good works
- **Preserved**: kept in faith until death & able to have assurance of faith
- **Glorified**: able to benefit from the ordinances of the church & be perfected at death

For a more detailed exposition of the 'Ordo Salutis' or 'Order of Salvation' there is a helpful article on the 'A Puritan's Mind'[9] website.

Remembering and repeating to ourselves often, in prayer, in praise, all that the LORD has done for us, all He has given us, all that He has saved us from will help us to see our current difficulties in a different light. The light of the hope and assurance that God, who has already done so much for us, will not abandon us now and is still, '**our refuge and strength, a very present help in trouble**'. Psalm 46:1 KJV

For some, trouble has been very present and very great throughout their lives. If you can look back over your life and see nothing but heartache, pain and loss, these truths are still for you. For, after all, here you are, reading this book, seeking help from the LORD for your difficulties. Providence may have been very hard, but you are still here. The LORD has brought you to this point, this time, this opportunity to find hope and light in your darkness. Cry with David:

> To the chief Musician, A Psalm of David.
> How long wilt thou forget me, O LORD? for ever? how long wilt thou hide thy face from me?
> How long shall I take counsel in my soul, having sorrow in my heart daily? how long shall mine enemy be exalted over me?
> Consider and hear me, O LORD my God: lighten mine eyes, lest I sleep the sleep of death;

> Lest mine enemy say, I have prevailed against him; and those that trouble me rejoice when I am moved.
> But I have trusted in thy mercy; my heart shall rejoice in thy salvation.
> I will sing unto the LORD, because he hath dealt bountifully with me.
> Psalm 13:1-6 KJV

You may not *feel* like the LORD has dealt bountifully with you but, in *fact* He has. He could have left you in your sins, destined for hell and a lost eternity. He has not. This fact alone is an inestimable mercy. Salvation, by itself, is the greatest gift any of us can be given. Your treasure is waiting for you in heaven. Eternal glory, joy, and delight in the very presence of the King of glory is yours. No worldly peace, no material comforts can possibly compare with this.

> For what is a man profited, if he shall gain the whole world, and lose his own soul? or what shall a man give in exchange for his soul? Matthew 16:26 KJV

HOMEWORK

What has the LORD done for you? Use one of the Journal pages to write your testimony. Trace the ways in which the LORD put people and circumstances into your life which drew you to Him. When did you first hear the gospel? How did your salvation come about? What further examples of the LORD's mercy and loving-kindness can you remember? How have your trials and difficulties brought you nearer to the LORD?

PRAYER

Thanksgiving, praise, prayers of gratitude. Repentance for any bitterness or resentment you are holding on to, any sense of entitlement. Remember the LORD owes us nothing but has given us so much!

Journal

Journal

WHAT TIME I AM AFRAID I WILL TRUST IN THEE. PSALM 56:3

It is of the LORD's mercies that we are not consumed, because his compassions fail not. Lamentations 3:22 KJV

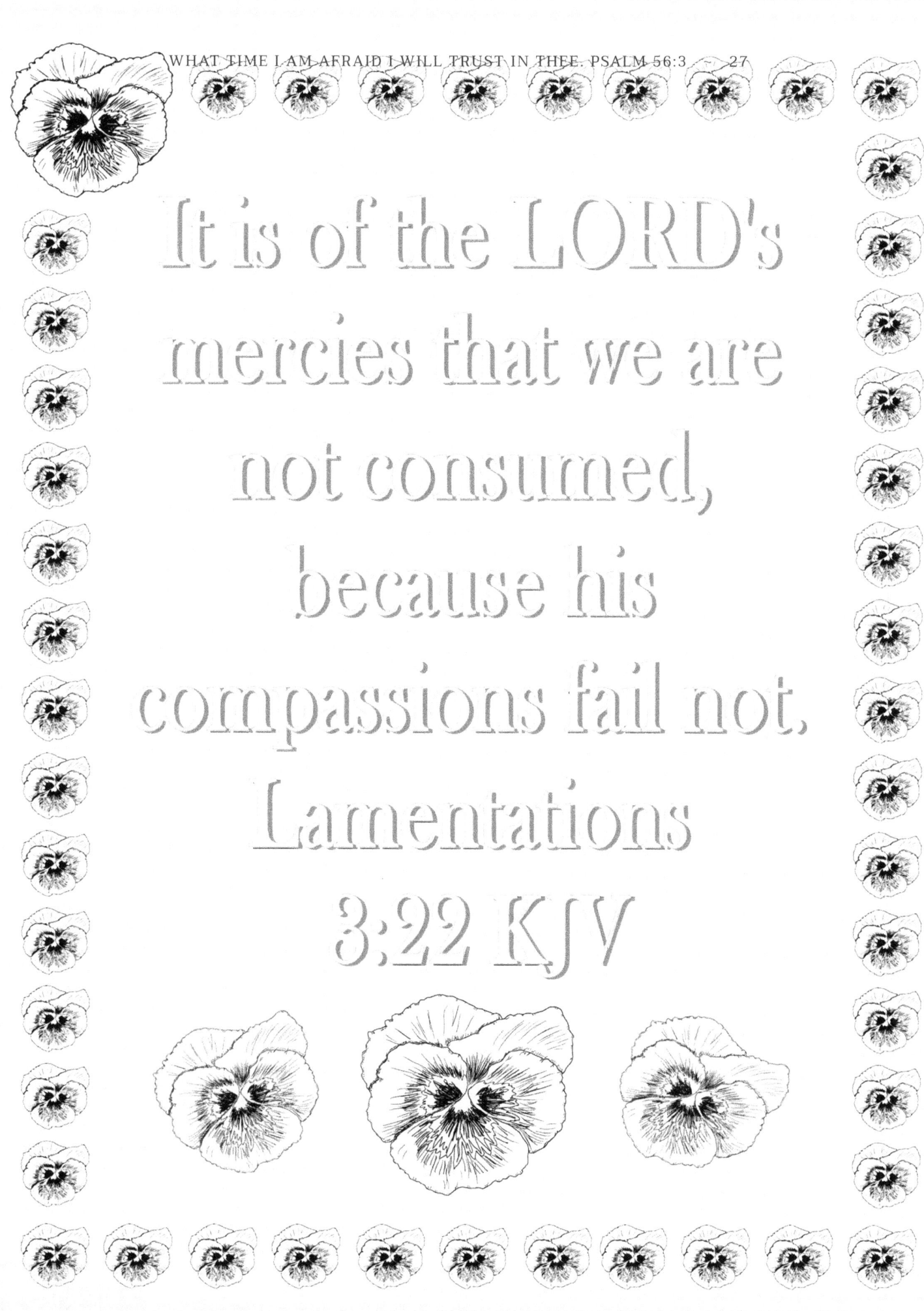

Chapter VII

Journaling : Bringing every thought into captivity

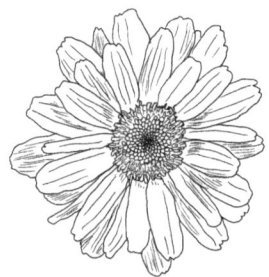
It would be helpful at this stage of your healing process to begin to use a journal. I have supplied some journal pages, but any blank notebook will do. The journal is not to record general events, thoughts, or past reflections, it is an accompaniment to this workbook. The first task is to begin to track and 'capture' your anxiety producing thoughts.

To begin with, you may not even be aware of many of these kinds of thoughts but, as you get more used to observing the way your mind thinks, they will become clearer.

Start with capturing those old thoughts about the LORD which are unbiblical and habitual. Like weeds, they take a while to root out but, when you spot them, challenge them, correct them in line with Scripture and ask for the LORD's help to bring them into captivity.

Next, focus on those habitual thoughts about yourself in relation to God which are faulty and unbiblical. A good way to notice these is to spot when you are talking to yourself in ways that you would not articulate out loud or would not use to speak about a loved one. We can often be mean and derogatory in the way we speak to ourselves. This is not helpful or productive. It is good to be honest and realistic, "I over-reacted to that. I didn't need to be so worried after all. I assumed the worst before thinking it through..." But not, "I'm a complete idiot! Why did I bother? What a fool I've been!" Can you see the difference?

If our 'self-talk' is full of emotional outbursts (albeit in our heads), derogatory and harshly judgmental, then we are speaking from our feelings not from an objective assessment of the situation. Accurate, truthful, objective assessment is what we should be moving towards. If we have committed sin, we should name it, confess it, repent, and receive the forgiveness of the LORD, seeking to avoid repeating that sin if possible, but we should not assume ourselves to be always at fault unless evidence supports it, or condemn ourselves as useless and hopeless. This is to fall into one of Satan's snares and speak falsehoods which deny the power and truth of what the LORD Jesus has done for us and in us.

People who suffer from anxiety are rarely so full of positive self-esteem that they commit the sins of pride in an overt manner, "How great am I? What a star!" However, watch out for the more subtle version of pride that comes with perfectionism. "I should have done that better, I should have been at the top of the class, I ought to have finished earlier..." This is a strange kind of pride that causes us to operate as if there were a perfect version of ourselves that wouldn't sin or fall short, if only we tried harder. There needs to be a humble acceptance that we'll never be perfect, never 'good enough' in and of ourselves. Our self-worth is not to be found in ourselves but in the Lord Jesus Christ in us. We have value because the LORD has set His love upon us and redeemed us *despite* ourselves! We are not 'works religionists', we are sinners saved by grace.

So, in your capturing of your thoughts, begin to track where and whether they are:

> A) Emotion-led
> B) Harshly judgmental
> C) Unrealistic (perfectionism)
> D) Exaggerated (use of absolutes – 'always', 'never', 'every' etc.)
> E) Catastrophizing (jumping to the worst-case scenario)
> F) Bitter and resentful
> G) Covetous
> H) Defeatist / pessimistic
> I) Assuming that God is not interested in us or even 'has it in for us!'
> J) Assuming the truths of Scripture are all very well in theory but have no practical application in our situation.

Your journal will not necessarily record what you do each day, but it should record events or circumstances that give rise to anxiety or increase the anxiety within you.

Spotting the 'triggers' that set you off can be very revealing. Often it is seemingly insignificant things that form triggers which set off a train of anxious thought.

A certain aroma (smell is particularly memorable when linked with important life events), a sound or music track, the way someone says something, they way the dishwasher has been stacked or clothes left on the floor, a scratch on the car, a family visit or myriad of other 'ordinary' things. Many small things can unwittingly become symbolic to us of larger, more troubling things. When we can spot and record these, we can begin to analyse the data, patterns and connections that are formed in our minds and which then feed through to our emotions, firing off our anxiety.

When you understand your own thought-life better, it becomes easier to see where challenges and changes can be made, where sinful or erroneous thoughts can be corrected, where conversations with those around us need to be had, reconciliation sought, different life choices made, and where we can better conform ourselves to God's will and way of living, with the wisdom, help and strength of the Holy Spirit.

> Journal entry examples:
>
> - The cupboard under the stairs got me again. I opened it, the broom hit me in the face, and I burst into tears! What a failure I am! I never seem to get through all the jobs I have on my list. I'm so inefficient!
> - Stubbed my toe on the end of the bed and said, "stupid woman" under my breath.
> - "Stop that, you fool!" I thought to myself as I caught myself chewing my lip again.
> - Worrying about what was going to happen at the GP next week. What will my test results show? What if it's bad news? What a worry wart!
> - Looking at the clock every minute and wondering why my husband isn't home yet. Has he had an accident? He always tells me if he's going to be late. He's been run off the road and is lying in a ditch somewhere! No, I am just being silly.
> - Can't stop thinking about what my friend said the other day. Did she really mean it? Should I ring her and talk it through? Am I making a mountain out of a molehill? This knot in my stomach doesn't seem to want to go away. Is it worry or is it something worse?

1) Highlight all the different names this person calls themselves in the above examples.

2) What effect do you think the name-calling has upon them?

3) What kinds of thoughts can you identify from the list above? List the letters (A – J)

These are not great life-changing incidents. They are small ordinary events that might happen many times in a day or week. However, the drip-feed of emotion-led negativity has a depressing and undermining effect. The way we order our thoughts, respond to situations, and treat ourselves in those situations, can help to lift us out of anxiety or plunge us deeper into it. Here is the remedy:

> **Casting down imaginations, and every high thing that exalteth itself against the knowledge of God, and bringing into captivity every thought to the obedience of Christ; 2 Corinthians 10:5 KJV**

Having taken the thoughts captive (writing them in the journal), let's bring them into 'the obedience of Christ'. We can do this by taking out the imaginary and emotional elements and seeing the truth objectively.

First 'capture':
The cupboard under the stairs got me again. I opened it, the broom hit me in the face, and I burst into tears! What a failure I am! I never seem to get through all the jobs I have on my list. I'm so inefficient!

Reframed factually:
The cupboard under the stairs did not 'get me'. It is not alive and has no malicious intent towards me. It does need reorganizing and tidying. Until I can get around to it, I must accept things are going to fall out on me. I need to

> decide if it's a priority compared to the other things I have to do. Being hit by a falling broom does not mean I am a failure. It just means the cupboard is not optimal at the moment.

See if you can reframe the other journal entries. We are aiming to be honest and objective and extract the emotional language from each situation; to 'cast down imaginations'.

You may be wondering how the altering of language around these small incidents can possibly make a difference to the very big problems and situations you face which are contributing to anxiety.

The language we habitually use infuses emotion (or not) into situations and events. If we are carefully being truthful and accurate in our language, rather than using exaggerated, emotional, or complaining language, we can change our mood and attitude. Practising with the many small things will lead to a more considered approach to the big things. This principle of accurate truthfulness is found in the 9th Commandment (**Thou shalt not bear false witness...Exodus 20:16 KJV**). The Westminster Larger Catechism Q.143 – 145, is particularly helpful in opening up the need for truth and honest dealings with each other and with ourselves.

Consider a gardening metaphor: You have a flower border to weed. There are many weeds of various sizes from tiny to huge. The tiny weeds take very little effort to get rid of. Loosen the earth a little and they can be pulled up. Very soon you can see the rewards for your effort. The ground is looking tidier and, by keeping on top of these small weeds, you ensure they do not grow larger and more difficult. When you begin to tackle the bigger ones, you have a method in place, you have the experience with the small weeds to encourage you and, therefore, it doesn't seem so daunting a task.

HOMEWORK

Getting into the habit of 'digging up' (capturing) your little weeds (thoughts), re-framing them without the emotion or unnecessary speculation and exaggeration, and applying objectivity and truth, will give you the skills to deal with the larger and more troublesome thoughts that come with the more dramatic events of life. Noting these in your journal will reinforce the point and help you to remember which Scriptures you chose to apply.

PRAYER

Ask the LORD to bring these thoughts to mind, to help you spot the negativity, exaggeration, and emotive language and ask the Holy Spirit to bring to mind scriptural truths to put in their place.

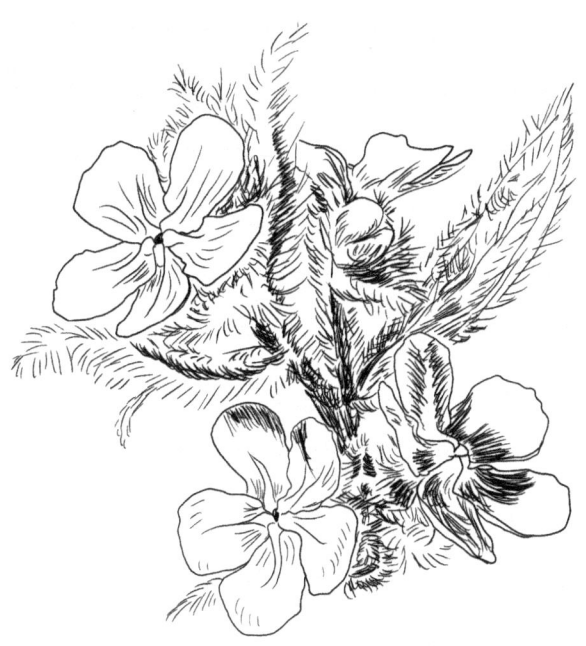

Journal

Journal

Chapter VIII

Renewing Your Mind

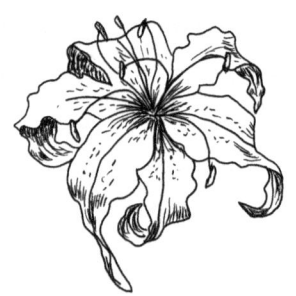

Another good use for your journal is to start collecting verses from Scripture that particularly speak to you and which you find helpful. You could start with any we have already quoted here that will help you to remember the practical aspects of your work and journey towards combatting anxiety.

Our unruly minds tend to frame things creatively, and sinfully in the light of human wisdom:

> Casting down imaginations, and every high thing that exalteth itself against the knowledge of God... 2 Corinthians 10:5 KJV

Rather than using that which is *against* the wisdom of God, we need to directly apply the Wisdom *of* God. We find that, of course, in the Word of God, the Bible.

Collecting helpful verses will form part of the process of renewing your mind. Learning Scriptures by heart, checking you have understood them in their context within a passage, reciting and applying them to everyday situations will help you to,

> Pray without ceasing. In every thing give thanks: for this is the will of God in Christ Jesus concerning you. 1 Thessalonians 5:17-18 KJV

When we mindfully apply Scripture and godly ways of thinking to the small everyday things, then we are building a foundation and defence which will give us courage and confidence to face the greater trials the LORD sends our way.

Identify those seemingly small things that give rise to a less than godly response, find a Scripture to apply to that thought, event or practice, and seek to transform your response and attitude into a truthful, objective, and godly one.

If you don't feel you know the Bible well enough to find relevant Scriptures, make it a key goal to read and know your Bible better. You can also use one of the many good Bible apps or desktop search engines to help you find relevant texts.

How many times have you read through the whole Bible? If you find focusing on reading difficult, how many times have you listened to an audio version? Knowing the Bible well will give you access to the richest resource you have available for spiritual and emotional healing and wellbeing. You will grow in confidence in the LORD and in His ability to forgive, restore, heal, guide, help, build you up in your faith and be your rock and hiding place.

Here is an example of applying mindful, godly thinking.

> Journal entry:
> Stubbed my toe on the end of the bed and said, "stupid woman" under my breath.
> Becomes:
> Stubbed my toe on the end of the bed and said, "Ooo, that hurt but nothing's broken. I can be thankful for that." And, **This is my comfort in my affliction: for thy word hath quickened me. Psalm 119:50 KJV**
>
> Journal entry:
> "Woke up with a cold. I can feel the dread rising. How am I going to cope with the day?"
> Becomes:
> "The Lord has sent me a cold bug. I wonder what He'll be teaching me through this? Patience, perseverance, trusting in Him to get me through the duties of the day?" **It is good for me that I have been afflicted; that I might learn thy statutes. Psalm 119:71 KJV**

When we train ourselves to have a heart of thankful praise by reciting Scripture and reminding ourselves of biblical truth and the true condition of things – God is Sovereign, ruling and reigning in righteousness, ordering all things for the good of His people – we begin to have a different mindset, a spiritually renewed mind, where we are no longer a prey to circumstance, battling alone in the world, but an heir of the household of God whom the LORD is sanctifying and fitting for eternal glory.

If we proactively train ourselves in the small, everyday and ordinary things of life, we will be arming ourselves with a renewed mind which is ready to cope with the greater afflictions and trials that the LORD may send us.

But how do I get there from here?

You may be thinking, "Journaling, learning Scripture, capturing thoughts, challenging what's true and what's false, what's feelings led, what's factual...that's all very well but I am struggling to get out of bed in the morning, let alone do anything that requires energy!"

If you have been finding anxiety so strong and difficult that you are wondering how you can possibly go forward from here, you may feel fragile and ready to break. You may feel broken already.

Let's look at our supreme example. How did the Lord Jesus Christ deal with the broken and lost? He attended to their bodily needs as well as spiritual needs. If they were hungry, he fed them, diseased, he healed them, and he taught them and forgave them. Let's look at your practical and bodily needs.

Do a brief life audit. Be factual not judgmental. For example, the answer to 'how many hours sleep you get' should not be 'not enough' or 'too much'. It should be 'around 6 hours' or 'an average of 8 hours'.

How much time / how often do you read the Bible and pray in a week?

How often do you get to church and / or prayer meeting?

How many meals a day to you eat?

What is your sugar, junk food, caffeine, and alcohol intake?

How many hours sleep do you get per night?

> What is your sleep/wake routine?
>
> How often do you keep your body/hair clean and tidy?
>
> How often do you do physical activity?
>
> How often do you have fellowship with any Christians during the week?

It is good to ask yourself these questions and see how near or far you are from doing any or all of these regularly. You may have circumstances which prevent you from being able to do some or most of these – looking after children, working shifts, financial pressures, demanding relationships, all of these and more. If your circumstances are such, then it is no surprise that you are stressed and anxious!

Write in your journal about why you are or are not able to do the things on the list. If there is one area that you could improve upon, what would it be? What do you think the most valuable area to improve would be?

Again, we look to our LORD for our example.

> Then said Jesus unto them, I will ask you one thing; Is it lawful on the sabbath days to do good, or to do evil? to save life, or to destroy it? And looking round about upon them all, he said unto the man, Stretch forth thy hand. And he did so: and his hand was restored whole as the other. And they were filled with madness; and communed one with another what they might do to Jesus. And it came to pass in those days, that he went out into a mountain to pray, and continued all night in prayer to God. Luke 6:9-12 KJV

Under pressure and threat from the Scribes and Pharisees who were looking for excuses to find accusations against Him, what does the LORD do? He prays to His heavenly Father all night!

When we are stressed, pressured, anxious, afraid: pray. If you can only get a couple of words out: pray. If you can only groan: pray.

> First things first:
>
> - Pray that the LORD will help you to pray.
> - If you are not eating regularly or enough to give your body energy, pray for the ability and will to eat, despite how the anxiety may be making you feel. Conversely, if you are eating or otherwise consuming substances that are reducing you to incapacity, pray for the ability to have self-control and only eat and consume what is necessary for bodily health. Self-medicating with alcohol or other substances will not help.
> - Pray that the LORD will give you such a love and desire for Him and His Word that you will make time to both pray and read Scripture every day.
> - Pray for the will and ability to get up, washed and dressed every day.
> - Pray that the LORD will enable you to attend the means of grace, the services and prayer meetings at church and have fellowship with Christians.
> - Pray for opportunities to be physically active.
> - Pray that the LORD will grant you better sleep.

Work towards these basic minimums looking to and depending on the LORD to help and give strength but knowing that you must do the actions. They are not going to happen to you. You must initiate. You must address the LORD in prayer and reach out to Him. The psalmist cried out,

> Hear my prayer, O LORD, and let my cry come unto thee. Psalm 102:1 KJV

Set yourself up a prayer schedule and mark off each day of the week. Remember, the length of time praying is not as important as actually praying. Better to pray for a minute a day than not pray at all! You can always improve and expand but, if you set yourself too ambitious a target, you are more likely to stop altogether.

WHAT TIME I AM AFRAID I WILL TRUST IN THEE PSALMS 56:3

Journal

Chapter IX

But I can't!

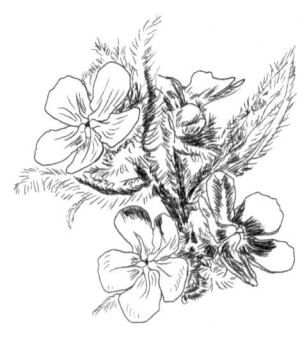

Healing from anxiety does not come as an instant cure and cannot be applied to you externally. You must make a commitment to work towards your own healing with the Lord's help. It begins with being willing to take the first step.

For some this has become incredibly difficult and even unattractive. In our sinful way of thinking, ducking out, being 'too ill' to do anything for ourselves, avoiding all responsibility, has become the most attractive option. Vegetating indoors, in our night clothes or under the duvet can feel 'safe' and non-threatening. However, it is a trap and a dangerous one at that.

I am not talking about the occasional retreat from everything challenging to have a restorative rest before 'girding up your loins' to carry on. I am talking about the, "I can't" way of thinking that leads us to a supposed incapacity where we have convinced ourselves that life is just too difficult and we are not up to the challenge, so our only option is retreat and inaction.

This supposed withdrawal into safety is, in fact, a threat to you which robs you of all joy, freedom, growth, development, or exhibiting of the fruit of the Spirit. It is a denial of faith and a belief that anxiety and fear is stronger than you are. It is not. The truth is that you, as a Christian, with the LORD's help, can overcome – but you must want to. You have to be willing to work, to suffer and to labour to overcome but then you will be able to say:

> For by thee I have run through a troop; and by my God have I leaped over a wall. Psalm 18:29 KJV

You don't need to believe in yourself or try and muster up strength from within. Rather, you need to believe in the LORD God Almighty, for whom nothing is impossible and who has power and strength to give to you when you have none of your own.

Let's look at Moses. We may think of Moses as a mighty man of God but he was not feeling very mighty when the Lord called him to go back to Egypt and head up the campaign to free the Hebrews from slavery. Moses complained,

> Who am I, that I should go to Pharaoh? Exodus 3:11 KJV, But, behold they will not believe me, Exodus 4:1 KJV, O my Lord, I am not eloquent…Exodus 4:10 KJV

This sounds very much like, "But I can't!"

Full of anxious fear, Moses was eventually only persuaded to go with Aaron as his mouthpiece. It was the LORD God who enabled and equipped Moses for the task ahead of him and by the end of his service to the LORD we read of him,

> And Moses was an hundred and twenty years old when he died: his eye was not dim, nor his natural force abated. Deuteronomy 34:7 KJV

This is not the description of a man consumed by the anxiety with which he began his pilgrimage! So how did this transformation take place? Step by step, day by day, year by year of faithful obedience and, in turn, the LORD enabling, equipping, empowering, and supporting him.

When we try to look within to our own resources, we will inevitably come up short. If anxiety has got such a hold on you that you are trying to hide from everything that feels the least bit threatening, then you have already tried and failed to find strength within to combat the fear. Stop looking inward and look upward. Look up to our great God, our awesome Creator, our loving heavenly Father, the KING OF KINGS AND LORD OF LORDS. He has the power to overcome all your fear. He can enable you to do that which, by yourself, you could never do!

> I can do all things through Christ which strengtheneth me. Philippians 4:13 KJV

If what you are doing is seeking to do the LORD's will in your life, then you will be strengthened to do it.

One prayer, one foot on the floor, one look at the Saviour rather than yourself. Begin.

In your journal, write down all the 'I can't' statements you have noticed yourself making. There may be 'It's too hard' thoughts or, 'I just feel too scared' or similar. Try and capture all these kinds of thoughts. There are probably links between these kinds of thoughts and certain activities which feel too challenging at the moment.

Try and analyse these thoughts and ask yourself:

- Have I been able to do this in the past?
- Do I have the skill or ability to do this, but I am questioning and doubting that?
- Is a past experience of difficulty relating to this activity dominating my thinking?
- Is the fear I feel when I think of doing this actually related to the activity or to the perceived effort involved in even attempting it?
- Is embarrassment over how it went last time overshadowing the thought of doing it again?
- Am I assessing my ability from my emotions or actual capacity?
- Is what I am trying to do in the LORD's will?

Which of the thoughts on your list do you *feel* or *believe* you can't do? Which are you afraid to do?

So now, list the ones that, if you were no longer afraid, you would be able to do. Which ones would you have the capacity to do, because you do have the skill or experience, if other thoughts and feelings were not getting in the way? Which are in line with God's will?

If you are not sure whether something is 'in the LORD's will' or not, don't look to your feelings on the matter.

Instead ask yourself:

> - Is it something we are commanded to do in Scripture? (Knowing Scripture well so that you can contextualize God's law and teachings, rather than lifting out 'proof texts' without context, is important.)
> - Is it something we are commanded not to do in Scripture?
> - If it doesn't seem obvious from Scripture, consider the effect or outcome of doing that thing – will that result in personal sin, harm to others, poor witness?

(For a helpful article on this subject, read "Decerning God's Will" by Sinclair Ferguson[10])

HOMEWORK

- Continue to collect and capture your thoughts and reframe them according to a godly way of responding.
- See if you can spot typical or repetitive thoughts and reactions which need to be reframed in a Biblical manner.
- Review some of the pages you have read so far. Spend time learning the Scriptures and colouring in the margins and pictures in a meditative manner.
- If this section has been particularly pertinent to you, go back to the beginning of this book and re-read the sections about the Sovereignty of God. Whatever you feel you lack, it is in the LORD that you will find that need met. Focus on facts and truth, not feelings.

PRAYER

- Practice praising the LORD and thanking Him for all His goodness and mercy.

- Praise the LORD for His Sovereignty, for His great love toward sinners demonstrated in the life, death, resurrection and ascension of our Saviour Jesus Christ.

- Pray for the LORD to help you and give you the strength to overcome your fears.

Journal

Journal

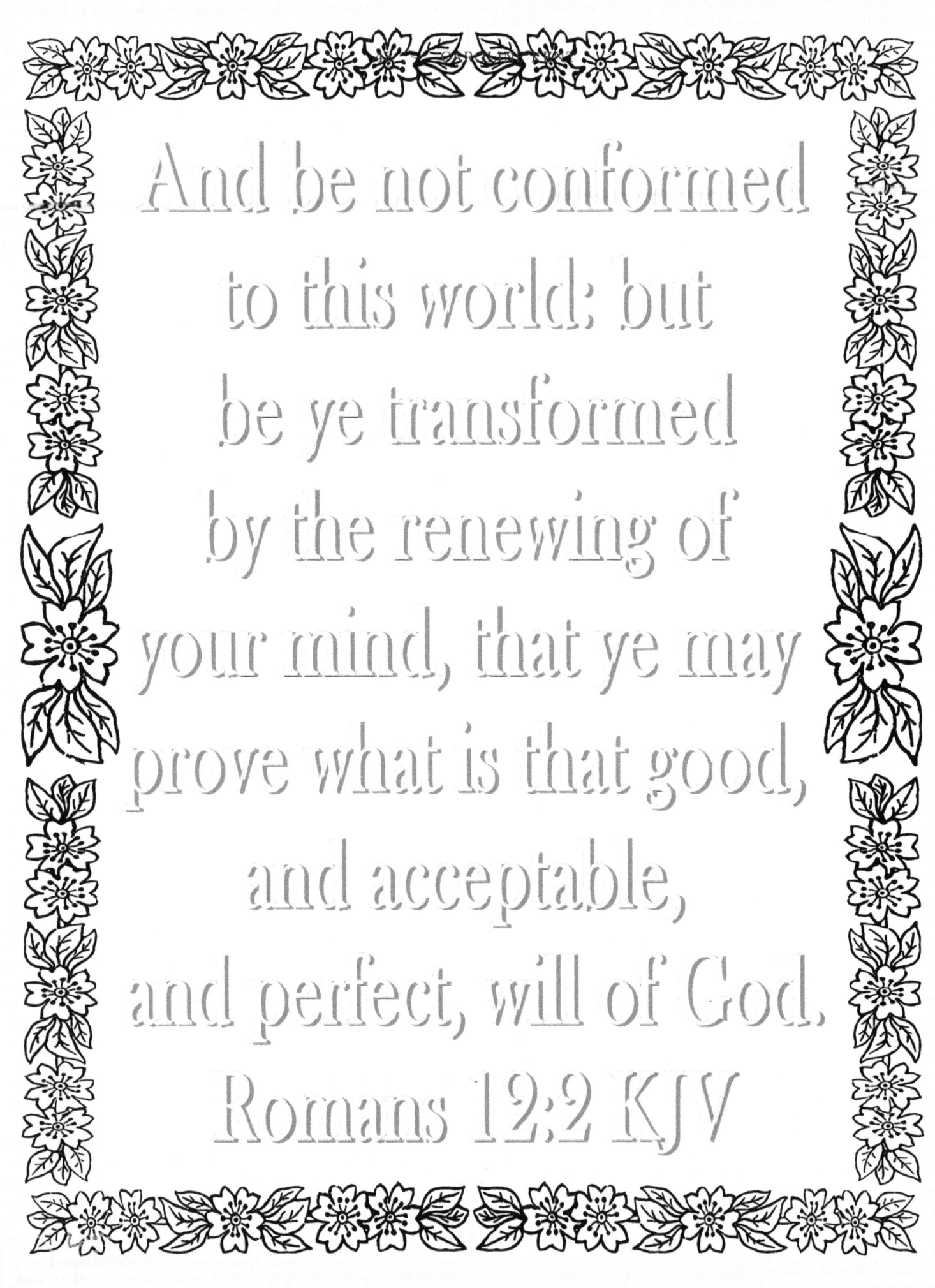

Chapter X

Fuelling Fear

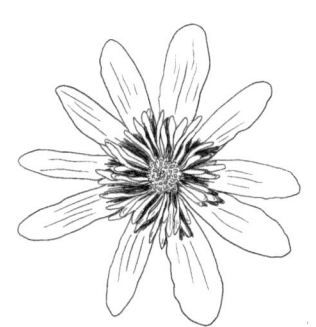

When we have been in a state of anxiety for a while, the very way we think fuels our fear. Which of course, in turn, keeps those horrible anxious feelings burning. There are certain kinds of thoughts which are prevalent:

- **Catastrophizing**: leaping to the worst-case scenario as if that is the only possible outcome of a situation and ignoring all the other, less drastic possibilities
- **Self-doubt**: undermining yourself and telling yourself negative things about your ability to do things or cope with the situation
- **Fortune telling**: imagining that you know the outcome without a doubt and acting upon your prediction regardless of whether it is accurate or realistic.
- **Running scenarios**: asking multiple 'what if?' questions and exploring all sorts of possibilities repeatedly. 'But what if this? Or what if that? But then this could happen. But then that could happen.' Restlessly with no resolution to the questions.
- **Mind reading**: assuming you know what other people are thinking (especially about you) without any evidence, and assuming it is judgmental and derogatory.

Don't worry if you have these kinds of thoughts, you are in good company! Let's look at some examples from Scripture:

Jacob, remembering his grief over the loss of Joseph, is fearful about letting Benjamin go into Egypt. He protests to his other sons,

> ...if mischief befall him by the way in the which ye go, then shall ye bring down my grey hairs with sorrow to the grave. Genesis 42:38 KJV

He has good reason to be anxious, but he is catastrophizing and fortune-telling. He doesn't know the outcome of sending Benjamin to Egypt with his brothers, but he predicts his own death as a result of 'mischief befalling' Benjamin. He is speaking from his fears, from his grief over Joseph, and assuming the worst. But what *doesn't* he do?

He doesn't pray to the LORD for wisdom and guidance in this matter. He doesn't look at the evidence (the other brothers have been to Egypt and back with no harm coming to them). He doesn't consider the promises of God about his family given to Abraham:

> That in blessing I will bless thee, and in multiplying I will multiply thy seed as the stars of the heaven, and as the sand which is upon the sea shore; and thy seed shall possess the gate of his enemies; Genesis 22:17 KJV

He could have used these things to reassure himself and could have been more at peace about sending Benjamin.

Elijah let his fears overtake him when Jezebel threatened his life (1 Kings 19:2). He was so dejected that he went into the wilderness and sat down under a juniper tree,

> ...and he requested for himself that he might die. 1 Kings 19:4 KJV

And this was immediately after that dramatic display of the power of God over the false prophets of the false god Baal! Why did he do this?

No doubt he was tired after the big day he had had, slaying false prophets, praying for rain after the long drought, and running to Jezreel. But why did he take fright at Jezebel's threat? Did he think God would let her slay him?

Out of his tiredness and sadness at the wicked response of Jezebel, Elijah thought and reacted emotionally. He forgot to think of all that God had just done, all that God was capable of doing, and he thought about his own weakness and assumed the worst:

> ...It is enough; now, O LORD, take away my life; for I *am* not better than my fathers. 1 Kings 19:4 KJV

Physical and mental exhaustion can seriously warp our responses and assessment of situations. Elijah couldn't imagine himself doing anything else. He couldn't imagine how he would muster the strength to fight off Jezebel. He forgot that he didn't have to.

There in the wilderness, the LORD let him sleep, sent an angel to bring him miraculous food to strengthen him and water to refresh him. In the strength of that food, he was enabled to travel forty days and nights until he came to mount Horeb. The LORD confounded Elijah's fears and pessimistic predictions and gave him the blessing of an encounter with Himself which gave him a new perspective. Something he had neither imagined nor predicted. There is a reason that we are not able to see into the future. We are supposed to trust our future to the LORD and seek His help when we are lost, exhausted, dejected and don't know where to turn. He *does* know where we should turn!

> Whither shall I go from thy spirit? or whither shall I flee from thy presence? If I ascend up into heaven, thou art there: if I make my bed in hell, behold, thou art there. If I take the wings of the morning, and dwell in the uttermost parts of the sea; Even there shall thy hand lead me, and thy right hand shall hold me. Psalm 139:7-10 KJV

The Psalmist reassures himself by thinking about who the LORD is and His wonderful attributes. We can each learn to do this. In our crisis moments, when our mind is doing summersaults and coming to wild and frightening conclusions, or it's just going round and round in an endless loop, we should stop. Breathe. Reach out to the LORD in prayer and remind ourselves that He is sovereign, mighty, present, all wise and that He loves us!

So, capture these thoughts in your journal and, when you notice them happening, turn to the LORD straight away for wisdom, strength and help in your time of need. Then challenge and restructure those thoughts, factoring in the strength and enabling of the LORD.

Journal

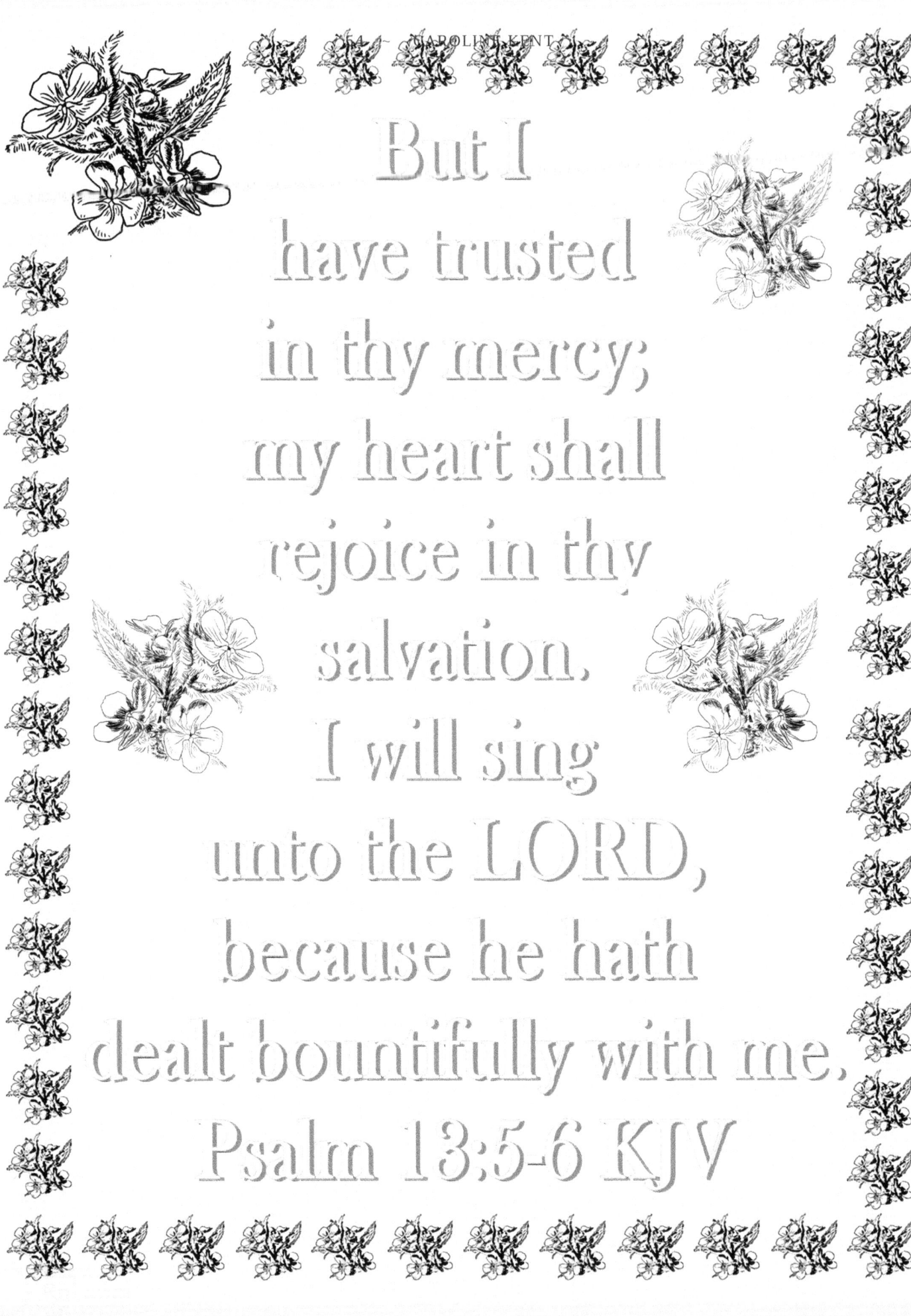

But I have trusted in thy mercy; my heart shall rejoice in thy salvation. I will sing unto the LORD, because he hath dealt bountifully with me.
Psalm 13:5-6 KJV

Chapter XI

Practicing a Peaceful Mind

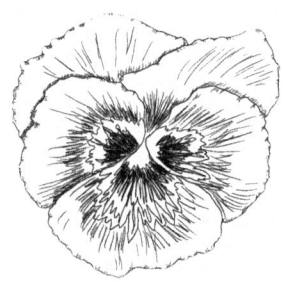

In the last section, we looked at some of the kinds of thoughts that the anxious mind can get caught up in thinking. Once you have learned to notice, catch, pray over, challenge and restructure those thoughts along scriptural lines, your focus should turn to the positive. Instead of letting the anxious thoughts flood your brain, you add good, wholesome, truthful, scriptural thoughts to your mind. Proactively filling your mind with biblical truth (learning verses, reading and re-reading the whole Bible, singing the psalms, reading sound Christian poems and trusted Bible study materials, and hearing faithful sermons) will give you precious wisdom to draw upon to combat the negative, self-focused, emotion-led and doubting tendencies.

> Be careful for nothing; but in every thing by prayer and supplication with thanksgiving let your requests be made known unto God. And the peace of God, which passeth all understanding, shall keep your hearts and minds through Christ Jesus. Finally, brethren, whatsoever things are true, whatsoever things are honest, whatsoever things are just, whatsoever things are pure, whatsoever things are lovely, whatsoever things are of good report; if there be any virtue, and if there be any praise, think on these things. Those things, which ye have both learned, and received, and heard, and seen in me, do: and the God of peace shall be with you. Philippians 4:6-9 KJV

The above passage is a treasure trove and road map for all godly minds, but especially for the anxious mind. Let's take each element:

Be careful for nothing

Our Lord Jesus Christ urged his disciples not to be those who are anxious and worried (Matthew 26:25-34). He reminds us, **Which of you by taking thought can add one cubit unto his stature?** I love this. The sheer effort of thinking, re-thinking and chewing over stuff that we cannot change is as pointless as screwing up all our energy and wishing we could make ourselves taller. If you can't change something, there is no point in expending any energy on it. "Easier said than done!" Yes, of course, but, not impossible. Worried about a loved one who is out of contact? You've tried all means of contact? You can do nothing else, but you CAN pray to the LORD God almighty who can do something (or rather, is already outworking His sovereign purposes in the matter). Expend your energy in prayer and put yourself in dependence upon the LORD to help you through the situation. Future things, tomorrow, can only be dealt with tomorrow. After you have done any reasonable preparation, then you have to wait—accept that fact.

In everything by prayer with supplication

So, in everything, prayer, asking the LORD for His wisdom, strength, help, guidance, and comfort. In everything, prayer. Everything. Prayer should be the first and continuous state of our minds. Connected to our loving heavenly Father and living 'Coram Deo': before the face of God. (R C Sproul)[11] Every moment of every day. When you know the LORD as your loving heavenly Father, you won't fear to live before the face of God, you'll want Him there, constantly.

Thanksgiving

Looking for things to be thankful for can be hard when you are bound up with anxiety but, there ARE always things to be thankful for when we look hard enough. We can thank the LORD we are still breathing, thank the LORD for the family and friends we do have, thank the LORD that it's a sunny day, thank the LORD the cat wasn't sick on the carpet just as you were leaving for work, thank the LORD that the kettle broke after you'd already made tea...

The point is that when we train ourselves to have an attitude of thanksgiving, we are not focusing on the negatives (be they real or imagined), we are looking at the truth, the facts, the present, the things we do have, not the things we don't.

We should, of course, be thankful that we are not headed for a lost eternity. Thankful that the LORD ever stirred us up to new life so that we might believe in Him (regardless of how wobbly we think that belief is). From the completely mundane to the heights of the spiritual mysteries of Salvation through Christ alone, we have multiple things to be thankful for at any given time. Proactively look for and find those things.

In your journal, keep a list of things you are thankful for. Read it often. Start your day thanking God for giving you a day in which you can think thankful thoughts!

Let your requests be made known to God

Anxious people can tend to be impatient people who make assumptions. Principally, they are impatient with themselves and assume that the LORD and everyone else is fed up with hearing their gripes. "God doesn't want to hear about my petty winging!", "My prayers are so pathetic!"

Let your requests be made known unto God. Tell Him everything. "But He already knows, so why bother?" Yes, He already knows everything before you even utter it. Prayer to the LORD is not about giving Him information. Prayer is relationship. When we openly and honestly pour out our hearts to the LORD about every little thing (and every big thing), we are entering into a relationship with Him where we are beginning to acknowledge that He hears us, cares about us, wants us to talk to Him in prayer and has provided the way, through the Lord Jesus, for us to have direct access to the throne of Grace. When we don't talk to the LORD in prayer, we are reinforcing the thought that we are alone and hopeless rather than the truth that we are never alone, and all our hope is found in Him.

And the peace of God, which passeth all understanding

Isn't one of the worst things about anxiety that lack of peace, that inner turmoil that seems never to end? Wouldn't you just love to have a sense of peace? Well, here it is, follow the steps above, practice them and the result will be peace. How? Because you will rest in the knowledge that the Sovereign LORD God of all the universe, who made you and everything else, who has decided to call you to be His child and knows all about your current worries, has you. He has you and your situation. He, who has the power that you don't, the strength that you lack, the wisdom you need, He has you. John Gill wrote

> *"...and underneath are the everlasting arms; that is, of God, which are the support of his people, and their protection, safety, and security; such as the arms of his everlasting love, which encircle them, and compass them about as a shield; his everlasting covenant, which is immovable, and in which they ever remain; eternal redemption and salvation, wrought out by Christ, which secures them from destruction; and everlasting power, by which they are kept and preserved as in a garrison; and everlasting consolation, which flows from all this: and so the arms of Christ, or his almighty power, are under the world, to uphold it in being; and under his church, to support it, on whose shoulders the government of it is; and under particular believers, whom he carries in his arms, embraces in his bosom, bears them up under all their afflictions and temptations, trials and exercises; nor will he ever suffer them to drop out of his arms, or to be plucked from thence..."* (Biblehub.com)[12]

This is the truth. How shall we not have peace?

The bodily feelings of anxiety are not telling you the truth, they are locking into habits, rehearsed many times but not reflecting reality. Even though you face an army of adversaries (be they thoughts or circumstances) it remains true that "underneath are the everlasting arms"! Grab hold of that truth, cherish it, repeat it, believe it, trust it. Drive out the anxious feeling and replace it with the shining truth of all that the LORD is and all He has done for His people.

Shall keep your hearts and minds through Christ Jesus

Remember, the peace that passes understanding, is God's peace. The peace of God. It is not something you or I can generate, it is something to be laid hold of that already exists. In the same way, the keeping of the Lord is already happening. In the wonderful high-priestly prayer of the Lord Jesus Christ the Lord prays,

> I pray for them: I pray not for the world, but for them which thou hast given me; for they are thine... Holy Father, keep through thine own name those whom thou hast given me, that they may be one, as we are. John 17:9-11 KJV

Shall the prayer of the Son to the Father be denied? No! So, through Christ Jesus, all his blood-bought children will be kept, and their hearts and minds would hardly be left out of that prayer.

Finally, brethren

Whatsoever things are true, honest, just, pure, lovely, of good report, having virtue, being praiseworthy, think on these things. [paraphrase]

When in an anxious state, what do you spend your time thinking about? When you are anxious, do you think about the last disaster, the next catastrophe, the embarrassment awaiting, the criticism looming? How does this make you feel?

But I can't help the thoughts that come into my head. Maybe not, but you can crowd them out so that they are stuffed in the corners!

Fill your mind with that which is righteous, lovely, beautiful, true and leave no room for the negative stuff. This takes effort. It is not going to happen by itself. An effort of will is required to shift the focus of your mind from those very easy, oh-so-natural negatives, and instead paint flowers, and colours and joy and happy memories and loving relationships and currant buns and rides in the countryside and worshipping the Lord in the beauty of holiness. Think on the Lord Jesus Christ! Choose to think on those good things over the dark, grey tones your mind throws up.

A good trick, when you are less anxious, is to write a list or make some colourful pages in your journal, with all the positive, true, scriptural, fun things you can think of so that, in your dark mood, you can turn to them and refocus your thoughts on the pure and virtuous things of God, and the delightful experiences of life that the LORD has enabled you to enjoy.

Those things, which ye have both learned, and received, and heard, and seen in me, do...

And the best antidote of all? Be salt and light. Do the commandments of Jesus. Love your enemies and your neighbours and your friends. Be and embody the teachings of Christ, as much as you possibly can, the Lord enabling you. Don't hide away from the life that the LORD has given you. Don't absent yourself from your family, your church, your obligations, your service. Do.

These words were spoken by Paul, under the inspiration of the Holy Spirit. Paul, more than most, had a right to feel anxious, traumatized, ready to hide from the world and huddle rocking in a corner. He recounts his experiences to the church at Corinth,

> In journeyings often, in perils of waters, in perils of robbers, in perils by mine own countrymen, in perils by the heathen, in perils in the city, in

> perils in the wilderness, in perils in the sea, in perils among false brethren; 2 Corinthians 11:26 KJV

Yet, the very same man says, **Be careful (anxious) for nothing**...Philippians 4:6 KJV

How? Yes, it is true, he was appointed by the Lord to be an apostle and therefore equipped for the task but, he was not made superhuman. He did have his personal struggles (Romans 7) and afflictions (2 Corinthians 12). How could he face all those things and carry on? **I can do all things through Christ which strengtheneth me. Philippians 4:13 KJV**. He kept his eye on and his trust in Christ Jesus, his LORD. He rehearsed the truths of Scripture and the promises of God. He praised the LORD in prison cells and trusted the LORD when all evidence might suggest shipwreck loomed (Acts 27).

"But Paul didn't seem to be an anxious type." Paul, as Saul, spent the first part of his life seeking to do the will of God but looking to his own strength. Was he misguided? Yes! But when the LORD opened his eyes and transformed him into a believer and an apostle, he instead, had his eyes up unto God. In that mental posture, the world looks a very different place. If you trust that God is in control and that in Him is found everything good, true and worthy of your attention, the dross of this world can be seen for what it is.

Whatsoever things are true...think on these things...those things you have seen in me, do.

> **And the God of peace shall be with you. Philippians 4:9 KJV**

HOMEWORK

Make a list of all the good things in your life for which you can be thankful. Practise reminding yourself who God really is (a true biblical understanding) and the knowledge that He is ever present with you.

Talk to the LORD, keep the dialogue going, remember that the LORD Jesus has provided you with access to the throne room of grace and covered you with His righteousness so that you are welcomed and accepted in His name.

Remind yourself that God is Sovereign
Praise the LORD often!

PRAYER

    Pray for the LORD to give you a peaceful heart and mind as you trust Him, dwell upon His excellencies and fill your mind with precious thoughts of Him.

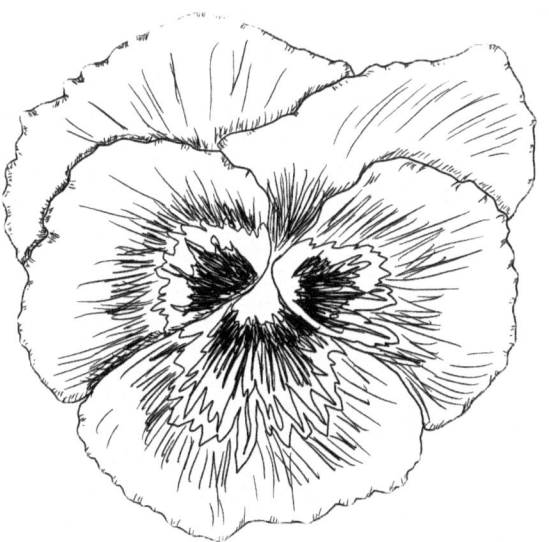

Journal

WHAT TIME I AM AFRAID I WILL TRUST IN THEE PSALM 56 vs 3

Journal

Chapter XII

Treating the Anxious Body

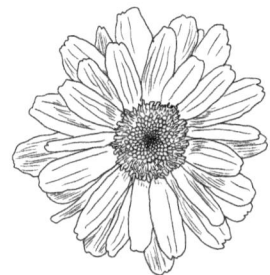
We are not disembodied souls. The Lord has given us a body and it is not a separate 'part' of us. We are integrated with our bodies. One of the most difficult aspects of anxiety is the horrible bodily sensations that come with it. Anxious thoughts are not only in the mind, they impact the whole body, and in many ways. The Psalmist captures some of this in **Psalm 102:**

> For my days are consumed like smoke, and my bones are burned as an hearth. My heart is smitten, and withered like grass; so that I forget to eat my bread. By reason of the voice of my groaning my bones cleave to my skin. Psalm 102:3-5 KJV

What we often don't realize is the strength of the connection between mind and body when it comes to anxiety and that, whether or not the circumstances which brought about the anxiety are still current, we *can* do something to alleviate the physical aspects of anxiety.

Breathing

Firstly, deep breathing. Before you leap back in horror, protesting that deep breathing is a practice from eastern religion, read on and see that deep breathing is simply a God-given method of helping ourselves to heal and recover from anxiety.

> And the LORD God formed man of the dust of the ground, and breathed

> into his nostrils the breath of life; and man became a living soul. Genesis 2:7 KJV

Now the LORD created man and woman with lungs to breathe in oxygen and to breath out carbon-dioxide. He also made them with a capacity to hold around 6 litres of air. However, many of us do not use this full capacity and, when we are anxious, we use even less. With tightness in the chest area, we snatch shallow breaths and put our respiratory system under stress. Short shallow breaths are associated, by the body and brain, with an alert of danger. Yet, for the person experiencing anxiety, the perceived danger may only be in their mind or may have passed a while ago. They are not in actual danger, but they are behaving as if they were, so the body stays in 'alert mode': tense, tight, shallow breathing.

Deep or (more accurately) diaphragmatic breathing (focusing on filling the lungs down to the diaphragm) draws in the full amount of oxygen per breath. This, in turn, is taken into the blood stream via the heart and the body experiences a quality infusion of oxygen. It is as if the body and brain receive an 'all is well' signal and begin to relax and feel like it is no longer in 'alert mode'. We are truly 'wonderfully made' (Psalm 139:14) by our wise Creator God!

Diaphragmatic breathing should be practiced regularly, at least three times a day for at least a minute. 3 minutes a day! You can do more and get more benefit, but just three minutes a day will begin to make a difference.

> So, sit up straight and imagine your arms are hanging off your shoulders in a relaxed way but your chest is in an open position. Place one hand just above your navel and under your breastbone. This is roughly where your diaphragm is to be found. It is a large muscle that sits under your lungs. Now, when you breathe in, do so through your nose but try to focus on filling the space above your hand so that your hand is pushed outward. This way you take in enough air to expand the bottom of your lungs. Once the bottom section is filled, focus on also filling the top section and you should feel your chest and rib cage expanding. Counting slowly to four may help as you do this. It can take a bit of practice if you haven't done it before. The key thing is not to scrunch up your shoulders, they should stay still and loose the whole time.
>
> Once you have mastered breathing in, we then focus on breathing out. Now you need to let out the air very slowly. The slower the better. Breathe out through your mouth but make a tiny hole, as if you were going to whistle, and

> slowly let the air out. Imagine you have blown up a balloon and now you are letting the air hiss out through the opening until the balloon is floppy.
>
> Got that? Now put the whole thing together, but with a pause in the middle.
>
> So, breathe in for a count of four, hold for a count of four, breath out for a count of eight (or more if you can manage it).
>
> - Breathing in 2,3,4
> - Hold 2,3,4
> - Breath out, 2,3,4,5,6,7,8....
>
> (You may feel just a little light-headed after this. That's fine, just don't try this while you are driving!)
>
> Rest for a moment and repeat. You may get three of four sets done in a minute.

The real benefit of practicing diaphragmatic breathing is felt when you build it regularly into your daily routine. Perhaps couple it with when you have a drink or a bathroom break, or before you move from one task to the next. A little but often will teach your body to be in a more relaxed and less tense state. Do it when you feel annoyed, upset, irritated. Do it before you go to sleep at night. The LORD gave you lungs with a 6-litre capacity. Use them! Remember, it is the LORD,

> **In whose hand is the soul of every living thing, and the breath of all mankind. Job 12:10 KJV**

Record your three minutes per day practicing diaphragmatic breathing.

Sunday	Monday	Tuesday	Wednesday	Thursday	Friday	Saturday
1 2 3	1 2 3	1 2 3	1 2 3	1 2 3	1 2 3	1 2 3

Moving

When we are anxious, we can forget to move our bodies. We can go into 'self-protection' mode: curled up, staying indoors and moving only for essentials. If we had previously been active, we may stop physical activity because of the crisis we are dealing with, or the illness we are enduring, or the fear of going out and being with other people. For all sorts of reasons, we can become less mobile when we are anxious.

If you can, running is really good for reducing the effects of anxiety. There are many instances of running in the Bible, some positive, some negative, the one that feels most applicable here is:

> **Which is as a bridegroom coming out of his chamber, and rejoiceth as a strong man to run a race. Psalm 19:5 KJV**

You may be neither a man nor a bridegroom but the image here is of joyful health, a man bursting with vitality who will enjoy running just because he can.

Vigorous exercise, which gets the heart pounding, stimulates the brain to release endorphins. These endorphins signal an 'I feel good' message to the brain which feeds through to the body. At the same time, while exercising, the body is using up adrenalin, a stress hormone, thus helping the body to feel more relaxed after exercise is over.

Those of us that have physical limitations can find getting vigorous, heart-pounding exercise difficult but still, we may be able to do the gentler kind of movement that, at least, stops us from seizing up altogether.

It can be tempting, as Christians, to forget that we have bodies and be so focused on the soul, spirit and mind that we neglect the body. Yet, the apostle Paul reminds us of our embodiment and the need to attend carefully, in a spiritual manner, to the needs of the body.

> **What? know ye not that your body is the temple of the Holy Ghost which is in you, which ye have of God, and ye are not your own? 1 Corinthians 6:19 KJV**

We must not drift into making it an idol, however! Christians should aim at being functional members of the body of Christ, not glistening jewels in the world's eyes. Physical health and fitness are useful, but should not be an end or aim in themselves.

Muscle Tension

When we have been anxious, stressed or on edge for a while, we build up tension in our muscles. Tightness around the neck and shoulders, lower back, chest, and abdomen are common. This muscle tension gives rise to aches and pains which just add to the misery! Investing a little time each day to ease these muscles will help to break down the effect of anxiety upon the body and send signals to the mind that we are not currently being threatened by physical danger, so we don't need to be ready to sprint to safety just at the moment.

(NOTE: If you are, in fact, under threat from physical assault, seek safety if possible! Do not stay in a situation where you are in physical danger. Escape to safety doesn't necessarily mean the end of a marriage or family, it can be the beginning of mending it, but do get outside help.)

So, how to ease muscle tension? With muscle tension! No seriously. A simple process of purposely tightening up the muscles that are already tight and then releasing them, can really help to reduce the tension.

For example, if your shoulders are tight and tense, scrunch them up as tight as you possibly can, whilst taking a deep breath in, and then release your breath and your shoulders at the same time. Do this a few times and notice the difference. Do this a few times a day and you will begin to break down the built-up tension. Do this before sleep in a methodical way from head to toe, tightening and releasing each muscle group in turn. Notice how much heavier you feel. This is the muscle in a more relaxed state. It's like when you pick up a sleeping child (dead weight) compared to a child who is awake and is holding itself up with muscles that are tense.

Another practical tip is to move your position on a regular basis. If you work at a desk, stand up every 30 minutes and stretch or walk about a little before carrying on. We can easily get 'set' if we sit still for too long and this contributes to the muscle tension and aches and pains, and the overall sense of not feeling well or coping. Reverse this with relaxing the muscles and moving them regularly and you'll get more of a sense that your body feels OK, and so you feel better and less anxious.

Moving more and stretching to relieve muscle tension will not, of course, change the circumstances that have caused your anxiety or cure the general sense of anxiety that you carry with you, but it will help alleviate some of the physical side effects.

Lots of little changes here and there can add up to a significant overall benefit. So don't ignore your body, look after it!

Do not use 1 Timothy 4:8 as an excuse to do nothing physical. Yes, physical exercise pales in comparison with the exercise of godliness but, it still profits us a little and to do a little of it every day will enable us to be more diligent in godly pursuits, since we'll have less bodily stiffness, pain or lethargy to overcome!

The Five Senses

One of the difficulties people with constant or frequent anxiety have, is that they have ceased to take much notice of current sensory input, and they are assuming input from the past or thoughts about the future to be giving them information upon which to operate.

The LORD has designed us with five senses: sight, hearing, touch smell, and taste. While we may not all have all of these, and certainly not all working to the same degree, we each do take in our information about the world through these senses. However, the 'am I safe?' mechanism is often skewed by non-sensory input.

A simple example. Imagine driving up to a set of traffic lights and slowing ready to stop. Person A eases to a stop and experiences no anxiety. Person B eases to a stop in exactly the same way but experiences a sharp pang of anxiety. There is no difference in the danger level. Both stop safely. Why does person B experience anxiety? Because a memory of having been rear-ended in the past, enters their mind and, in a moment, they re-experience the collision and even feel the pain they felt on the occasion. Memory has kicked in and non-sensory input has occurred.

When we have experienced events which have given rise to a high level of emotion or pain, we may easily be 'triggered' when in a situation that reminds us of the previous event, even if actual danger is not present. We remember the original event and prepare ourselves to cope with it all over again just in case history repeats itself. This is a helpful mechanism in learning, for which we can be thankful, because it means we are less likely to repeat damaging mistakes, and we learn to negotiate difficult or dangerous things through problem solving. The issue with anxiety is that this mechanism has gone into overdrive. It's called 'hypervigilance' and it is a state in which people are living as if danger is always imminent.

Of course, for some people, living with an abusive person, for example, the danger is constant and imminent, and learning how to live without that when the danger has finally passed takes time.

Thankfully, we have a God who heals and restores and transforms!

So, how can we move from re-living the past or fearing the future whilst missing the present and having the present spoiled by anxious thoughts and feelings?

Practice using the senses that the LORD has blessed us with. Use them purposefully and proactively to focus on the moment you are in and receive input from your senses.

Find a safe and comfortable place to sit. Take with you a small piece of food like a raisin or a nut (you'll need it in a minute). Now, you are going to purposefully experience input from each of your five senses in turn (to the extent you are able).

> **Sight**: pick a colour and, looking around the space that you are in (hopefully it's not a minimalistic white room!) see how many different examples of that colour and related shades and tones of it, you can see. Spend at least a minute doing this. Let your eyes explore and be curious about shapes, patterns, and textures you can also see. Thank the LORD for the vision that you have, if you have any. If you have lost your vision, or never had it, consider what it will be like in glory, to be able to see perfectly, and be thankful for that.
>
> **Hearing**: sit still and quiet and count how many different sounds you can hear. Do this for long enough to begin to hear the background sounds and notice those noises which you would not normally pay any attention to. Be thankful to the LORD for your hearing. If you do not have the capacity to hear, be thankful for the aid and helps available, sign language and subtitles. Again, consider what it will be like to hear perfectly in glory. To be able to hear the constant praise of our great God and His very voice speaking to you!
>
> **Touch**: use your fingers and hands to touch all the different textures within your reach. Your clothes, your skin, your hair, the seat you are on. Think about your body as it connects to the seat, the floor, the air around you. Feel the air across your skin under your nose as you breathe in and out. What does the air feel like on your tongue? Thank the LORD for the sense of touch and the ability to feel ourselves to be present and real.
>
> **Smell**: now think about what you can smell. You might think there is nothing to begin with but give it time. What does the air smell like? Dry, musty, humid, dusty, fragranced? Can you smell the last meal cooked, the washing soap on your clothes, your own scent or deodorant? Focus hard. Many people had their sense of smell impaired by the COVID-19 virus, but be thankful for what you can smell.
>
> **Taste**: now pick up the nut or raisin or small piece of food you chose. Begin by experiencing what it looks like, and what sound it makes (if any) as you move it between your fingers (I hope it's not too gooey!). What does it feel like

> in your fingers? What does it smell like? And finally, touch it to your tongue, take a small bite from it, roll that around and experience the flavour, chew and let the whole thing fill your mouth with flavour and sensation. When it is thoroughly chewed, swallow it and track what it feels like going down. Thank the LORD that you have food to eat and can make choices about flavour and between foods.

Hopefully, several things happened while you did this exercise:

- you gained a new appreciation for the senses that the LORD has blessed us with.
- you were so focused on doing the exercise that you got a little break from the anxieties and stress you have been experiencing.
- you feel very thankful to the LORD for all that He has given you that sustains you every day and enables you to function in the world.

Do this activity regularly to break yourself out of the anxiety cycle. The more you do it, the better at it you'll get and you'll see that living in the present can be quite different from every moment being overshadowed by the past or spoiled by a sense of doom about the future.

Practice the same mental attitude as you go about your business. To be present in that moment, thanking the LORD and feeling grateful for what is, rather than in fear of what was or might be.

Not your own

These bodies (and our souls), which form part of the larger body of the members of Christ, are not our own. They have been bought with a price. The infinitely high price of the Lord Jesus Christ's suffering and death on the cross. Therefore, we need to give them the care and respect we would give to any precious borrowed or loaned item. Taking healthy exercise, according to our ability, eating healthily and enjoying the bounty provided by the LORD (but not too much), resting ourselves from work and restoring our minds and spirits on the LORD's Day each week, patterning our lives around the helpful daily routines of prayer, Bible reading, eating, exercising, working, sleeping and then attendance at the means of grace whenever we can. Such structure helps to reduce anxiety as we experience ourselves 'plugged in' to the provisions that the LORD has made and ordained for our good, and experience the support that structure, fellowship and a regulated lifestyle gives us.

Have your routines gone to pot because of your anxiety? Perhaps you never had any routines? Do you do any exercise? Do you take any care to eat healthily? Do you make sensible provision for sleep and reserve the LORD's Day for worship and rest from work as far as possible?

When you think of your body as being 'on loan' from the LORD, rather than your own to do with as you wish, what thoughts arise in your mind? Do you struggle with this idea?

Explore this biblical truth.

> Ye are not your own. For ye are bought with a price: therefore glorify God in your body, and in your spirit, which are God's. 1 Corinthians 6:19b-20 KJV

Write about what you would do differently if you really understood that your body is the temple of the Holy Spirit and belongs to God, not you.

HOMEWORK
- Practise diaphragmatic breathing several times a day.
- Do some form of physical activity—as vigorous as you can for at least 5 minutes a day.
- Practise tensing and releasing those areas of tension in the body.
- Practise using the senses the LORD as given you to experience the present. Worship Him as you appreciate your surroundings.
- Treat your body well but don't worship it, worship the LORD who gave you this body and ask Him to help you with the circumstances of your life, for He gave you those too, in His sovereignty.

PRAYER

Pray these verses:

Be careful for nothing; but in every thing by prayer and supplication with thanksgiving let your requests be made known unto God. And the peace of God, which passeth all understanding, shall keep your hearts and minds through Christ Jesus. Philippians 4:6-7 KJV

WHAT TIME I AM AFRAID I WILL TRUST IN THEE PSALM 56 V 3

Journal

Journal

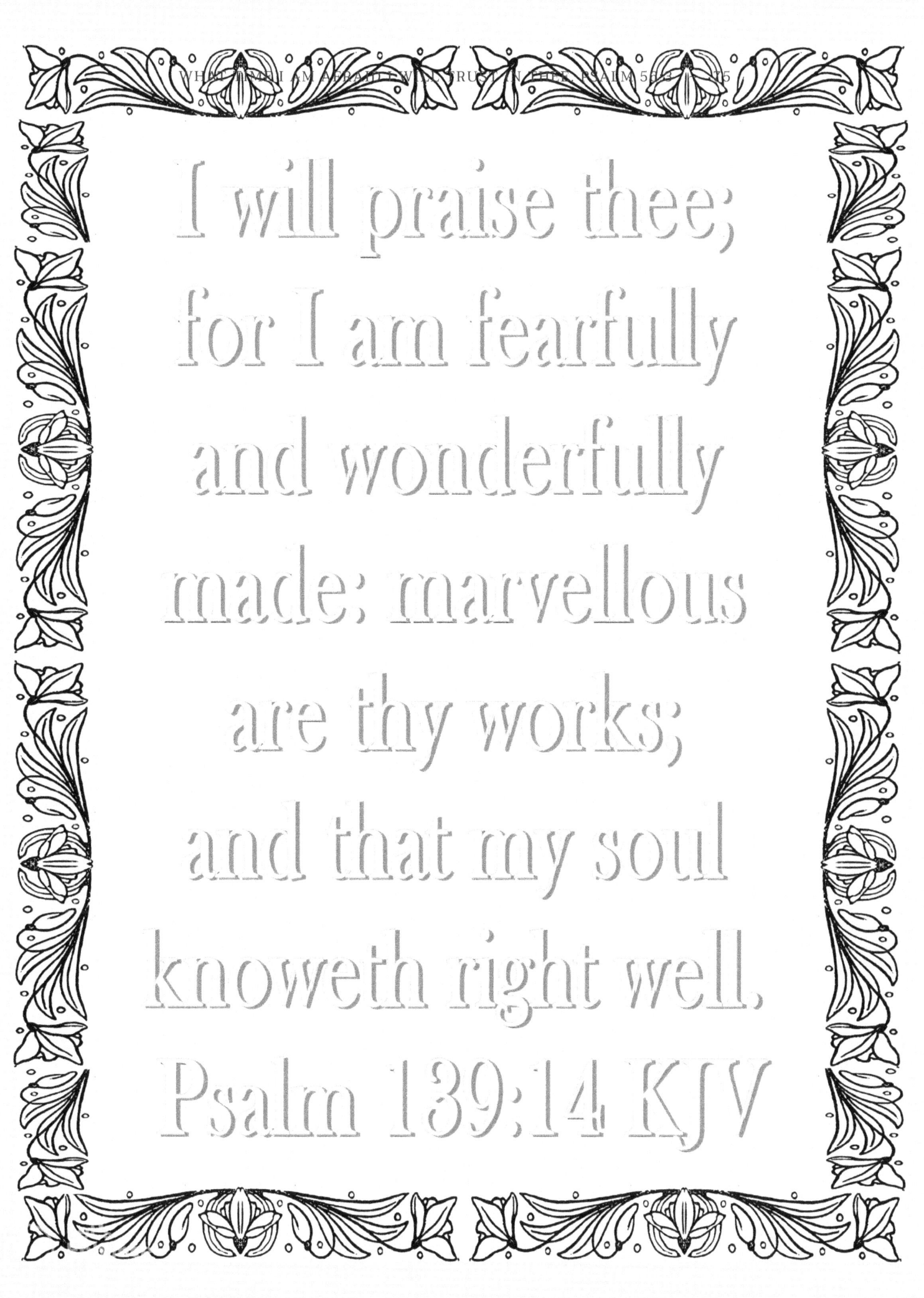

Chapter XIII

Conclusion

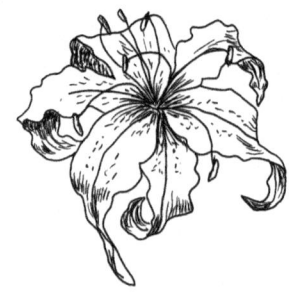
You have reached the end of this workbook. However, you have not finished the work! Changing automatic reactions, engrained thought patterns and habitual behaviours does not happen after reading through a book. It happens through repeatedly reading and doing the activities, through labouring and making a huge effort to turn your mind to a better, more godly way of thinking and therefore being.

The Bible is full of farming analogies and for good reason. The preparation of the ground—digging over, pulling out rocks and weeds, ploughing into straight furrows: hard work! The watering, weeding, watching and waiting for shoots to grow requires patience and perseverance. The harvest, though rewarding, doesn't come without heavy labour. So too, the renewing of the mind and the ability to trust the LORD and therefore experience less anxiety, is hard work! The rewards, however, are not just less anxiety, but, a closer walk with your God, a better understanding of your relationship with Him, a growing love and appreciation for all that He has done and is doing in and through you by His Holy Spirit.

One of the reasons this workbook has some decorative borders and colouring sheets, is to entice you to go back to colour the pages and think about the messages and teaching. To encourage you to read and re-read and meditate upon the guidance and the Scripture while you colour and, having poured in all that time and effort, to have a beautifully personalised manual to which you can refer in the future.

Human beings are slow learners. This has nothing to do with intelligence, we learn only slowly those lessons that are most vital to our walk with God because we battle against indwelling sin. We need to hear the Gospel and read our Bibles continuously because truth and wisdom seem to slip all too easily from our grasp in the face of daily life and all its challenges. Therefore, seeking the LORD's help, go back over this book again and again and do the tasks repeatedly.

Take heed of the warning of the LORD through Jeremiah:

> But this thing commanded I them, saying, Obey my voice, and I will be your God, and ye shall be my people: and walk ye in all the ways that I have commanded you, that it may be well unto you. But they hearkened not, nor inclined their ear, but walked in the counsels and in the imagination of their evil heart, and went backward, and not forward. Jeremiah 7:23-24 KJV

To escape the imagination of our evil hearts we must fix our eyes upon the Lord Jesus Christ, upon the unerring truths of the Bible and the wisdom that only the Holy Spirit imparts to the redeemed of the LORD.

Acknowledgements

I would like to thank the many counselling clients I have worked with over the years who have trusted me to hear their stories, given me insight into the thoughts and feelings experienced in the midst of anxiety, and who have been willing to put into practise the guidance from this book.

However, the LORD must have all the glory! His sovereign hand brought me into counselling, brings my clients to me and continues to guide and teach day by day. He sustains me and helps me and, many a time, an arrow prayer for wisdom from above has been wonderfully answered. It is a joy and privilege to share biblical truth with needy souls and to see it bare fruit.

I have benefitted hugely from reading the Puritans and could recommend a long list! To see those I have found helpful in the counselling context, please visit my website and see the 'Recommended Reading'[13] page.

This book forms a 'foundation' and I plan to produce additional material for those kinds of anxiety which have become more troublesome and deep routed than 'every-day' anxiety. I hope to produce a second volume which covers:

- Lack of assurance
- Blasphemous thoughts
- Religious scrupulosity
- Obsession, compulsions and rituals
- The unforgivable sin
- Prevarication
- Perfectionism

Caroline Kent

Bibliography

1. The Westminster Confession of Faith (Ligonier.org) https://www.ligonier.org/learn/articles/westminster-confession-faith
2. The Westminster Confession of Faith (Ligonier.org) https://www.ligonier.org/learn/articles/westminster-confession-faith
3. 1689 Baptist Confession https://www.the1689confession.com/
4. Arthur W Pink *The Sovereignty of God* - https://www.monergism.com/thethreshold/sdg/pink/sov2015_p.pdf
5. Arthur W Pink *The Attributes of God* - https://www.monergism.com/thethreshold/sdg/attributes_online.html
6. Monergism.com
7. John Gill (Biblehub.com) https://biblehub.com/commentaries/gill/psalms/139.htm
8. Matthew Henry (Biblehub.com) - https://biblehub.com/psalms/139-7.htm
9. 'A Puritan's Mind' - https://www.apuritansmind.com/tulip/ordo-salutis-the-order-of-salvation/
10. 'Decerning God's Will' by Sinclair Ferguson - https://www.monergism.com/discerning-gods-will
11. ''Coram Deo': before the face of God.' R C Sproul - https://www.ligonier.org/learn/articles/what-does-coram-deo-mean
12. John Gill (Biblehub.com) - https://biblehub.com/commentaries/deuteronomy/33-27.htm
13. Recommended Reading List - https://www.counselling-with-caroline.co.uk/recommended-reading

About the Author

Caroline has been married to Jeremy Kent since 1995 and together, the LORD has led them to Bentley Reformed Baptist Church where Jeremy is the Elder.

Caroline has a degree in theology, is a qualified teacher and counsellor and practises as a Biblical Counsellor from her home in Suffolk. The majority of her work is via internet video. She has been counselling people the length and breadth of the United Kingdom and abroad since 2011.

One of the reasons that Caroline changed from full time teaching to counselling was that she became unable to work full time due to the onset of Fibromyalgia, Arthritis and Chronic Fatigue in 1998. While this has been a struggle and frustration at times, it has also been a great blessing and Caroline can trace the hand of her Sovereign LORD God in sending this affliction. She has learned (and continues to learn) many valuable lessons personally, and her understanding of suffering has enabled her to have empathy with others in pain of all kinds.

Many of Caroline's clients come to her with anxiety, amongst other issues, and this book was born out of her experiences with treating over two hundred different individuals, her research into the Puritans with their practical, pastoral theology and, of course, Biblical studies and much prayer!

It is her hope that many will benefit from using this book.

Journal

Journal

Journal